Clinical Judgement and Decision Making in Nursing

Sara Miller McCune founded SAGE Publishing in 1965 to support the dissemination of usable knowledge and educate a global community. SAGE publishes more than 1000 journals and over 800 new books each year, spanning a wide range of subject areas. Our growing selection of library products includes archives, data, case studies and video. SAGE remains majority owned by our founder and after her lifetime will become owned by a charitable trust that secures the company's continued independence.

Los Angeles | London | New Delhi | Singapore | Washington DC | Melbourne

3rd Edition

Clinical Judgement and Decision Making in Nursing

Mooi Standing

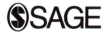

Los Angeles | London | New Delhi
Singapore | Washington DC | Melbourne

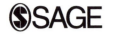

Learning Matters
An imprint of SAGE Publications Ltd
1 Oliver's Yard
55 City Road
London EC1Y 1SP

SAGE Publications Inc.
2455 Teller Road
Thousand Oaks, California 91320

SAGE Publications India Pvt Ltd
B 1/I 1 Mohan Cooperative Industrial Area
Mathura Road
New Delhi 110 044

SAGE Asia-Pacific Pte Ltd
3 Church Street
#10-04 Samsung Hub
Singapore 049483

Editor: Alex Clabburn
Development editor: Richenda Milton-Daws
Production controller: Chris Marke
Project management: Swales and Willis Ltd, Exeter, Devon
Marketing manager: Tamara Navaratnam
Cover design: Wendy Scott
Typeset by: C&M Digitals (P) Ltd, Chennai, India
Printed in the UK

First edition published 2011
Second edition published 2014
Third edition published 2017

Library of Congress Control Number: 2017931590

British Library Cataloguing in Publication data

A catalogue record for this book is available from the British Library

ISBN 978-1-4739-5725-1
ISBN 978-1-4739-5726-8 (pbk)

Contents

Transforming Nursing Practice is a series tailor-made for pre-registration student nurses. Each book in the series is:

- ○ Affordable
- ○ Mapped to the NMC Standards and Essential Skills Clusters
- ○ Full of active learning features
- ○ Focused on applying theory to practice

Each book addresses a core topic and has been carefully developed to be simple to use, quick to read and written in clear language.

> **"**
>
> An invaluable series of books that explicitly relates to the NMC standards. Each book covers a different topic that students need to explore in order to develop into a qualified nurse... I would recommend this series to all pre-registration nursing students whatever their field or year of study
>
> **Linda Robson**
> **Senior Lecturer, Edge Hill University**
>
> The set of books is an excellent resource for students. The series is small, easily portable and valuable. I use the whole set on a regular basis.
>
> **Fiona Davies**
> **Senior Nurse Lecturer, University of Derby**
>
> I recommend the SAGE/Learning Matters series to all my students as they are relevant and concise. Please keep up the good work.
>
> **Thomas Beary**
> **Senior Lecturer in Mental Health Nursing, University of Hertfordshire**
>
> **"**

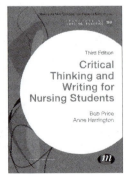

Third Edition
Critical
Thinking and
Writing for
Nursing Students

Bob Price
Anne Harrington

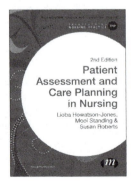

2nd Edition
Patient
Assessment and
Care Planning
in Nursing

Lioba Howatson-Jones,
Mooi Standing &
Susan Roberts

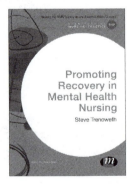

Promoting
Recovery in
Mental Health
Nursing

Steve Trenoweth

About the author

Dr Mooi Standing is an independent academic consultant with over 40 years' experience that includes: (i) practising mental health and adult nursing in a range of hospital and community settings; (ii) lecturing pre-registration and post-registration nursing students from certificate to Master's level and presenting scholarly papers at international nursing conferences; (iii) researching how nurses develop clinical decision-making skills and publishing articles, books and chapters on this topic for nursing students, registered nurses and advanced practitioners; and (iv) providing external consultancy in curriculum development and quality enhancement of nursing programmes both nationally and internationally.

Mooi is currently a Series Editor for Learning Matters/Sage's 'Transforming Nursing Practice' books, an accredited Nursing and Midwifery Council (NMC) Quality Assurance Reviewer of nursing educational programmes and a Professional Regulator as a Panellist on the NMC Practice Committee.

Acknowledgements

One of the important themes of this book is that good nursing care depends upon effective collaboration with others. It also applies to writing and I need to thank the following people.

I am indebted to my former students who took part in the research study which inspired and informed this book. I thank them for their openness and reflective, critical self-examination.

I could not have written the book without the infinite patience, rock-solid support, contribution in researching case studies and critical feedback of my beloved husband, Michael Standing.

I wish to dedicate this book to the late Professor Emeritus Ken Hammond, University of Colorado, for his precious time and generosity in encouraging me to apply cognitive continuum theory to nursing decisions.

I must express my gratitude and appreciation to my special friend 'Annie' (you know who you are!) for her selfless openness, honesty and generosity in sharing her observations and experiences as a patient in an acute hospital setting, and for giving me permission to use these for the three case studies in Chapter 12. Last but not least, it has been a pleasure to work with Learning Matters in writing this book, and I would like to express my thanks to Richenda Milton-Daws for her helping me be a little less verbose and more concise.

Dr Mooi Standing

Introduction

This introduction looks at who should read this book, what it is about, why it is important and how it is structured, and gives a brief overview of the NMC Standards and learning activities.

Who should read the book?

The main audience for this book are pre-registration nursing students of all levels, from beginner to finalist, in adult, mental health, child and learning disability pathways. It is also recommended for all registered nurses. It should interest clinical mentors and assessors who support students' work-based learning during their practice placements. Lecturers in nursing might find the book a helpful resource for relevant learning or teaching activities. Midwives may also be interested in applying the PERSON evaluation tool to practice.

What is it about?

The book draws together a wide range of knowledge, skills, attitudes and values that characterise safe and effective clinical judgement and decision-making in nursing. This includes looking at the numerous decisions nurses have to make, the variety of evidence and observations that inform clinical judgement and the different approaches to decision-making according to patients' varying needs, available resources and time constraints. Working through the book will help students to develop their understanding and competence in applying and evaluating clinical decision-making skills to give the best possible care.

Why is it important?

Learning about clinical judgement and decision-making is important because it makes us continually question whether our actions are beneficial to patients, and discover and apply better ways of caring for them. Nursing is a practice-based profession, and everything we do affects the health and wellbeing of those we care for. Nursing practice needs to be safe and effective in promoting health and recovery from illness, and in relieving suffering. Thus, nursing practice and actions need to be well-reasoned, responsive to individual needs and evidence-based as appropriate, and to have practical outcomes that benefit patients. We cannot achieve this without exercising sound clinical judgement and decision-making. We are also accountable for the quality of care we provide, and this requires us to explain, justify and defend clinical judgement and decision-making. Reading this book, looking at case studies and doing the activities will help you to integrate theory and practice in clinical judgement and decision-making. It will also help you to apply the required standards in *The Code* (NMC, 2015) to evaluate and improve decision-making and nursing care.

How is it structured?

The format reflects findings of a research study exploring nursing students' perceptions and experience of clinical decision-making skills from the beginning of their programme to the end of their first year as registered nurses. Ten perceptions or features of clinical decision-making were identified from the research and they provide the focus for Chapters 2–11.

Chapter 1 *What is clinical judgement and decision-making in nursing?* – clarifies terms and shows how all ten perceptions of clinical decision-making are applied to one person's care.

Chapter 2 *Collaborative clinical decision-making* – explores consultation, negotiation and co-operation skills with patients and other health professionals in delivering care.

Chapter 3 *Using observation to inform decisions* – emphasises the importance of what we see or hear as evidence about patients' physical or mental health to inform decisions.

Chapter 4 *Systematic clinical decision-making* – combines critical thinking and problem-solving skills to comprehensively assess, plan, deliver care, review and revise outcomes.

Chapter 5 *Standardised clinical decision-making* – looks at applying local NHS Trust policies and procedures and national evidence-based clinical guidelines to enhance care quality.

Chapter 6 *Prioritising decisions in delivering care* – shows how undertaking risk assessment and management informs how resources are targeted nationally and locally in healthcare.

Chapter 7 *Experience and intuition in decision-making* – looks at the way we accumulate a subconscious repertoire of knowledge and skills that we draw upon when events prompt us to do so.

Chapter 8 *Reflective judgement and decision-making* – helps you to consciously review personal, theoretical and practical understanding of a clinical situation as a guide to future action.

Chapter 9 *Ethical sensitivity in decision-making* – covers respect for patients' human rights of freedom of choice, informed consent, confidentiality and sensitivity in resolving ethical dilemmas.

Chapter 10 *Accountability for nursing decisions* – identifies who we are answerable to, how we are called to account and the importance of quality assuring standards of care.

Chapter 11 *Confidence in clinical decision-making* – helps you to develop self-assurance and professional assurance to inspire confidence in patients and team members that you can be trusted.

Chapter 12 *Matrix decision-making model and PERSON evaluation tool* – applies the ten perceptions of decision-making and conceptions of nursing in a new framework to guide and evaluate nursing decisions.

NMC Standards for Pre-registration Nursing Education and Essential Skills Clusters

The Nursing and Midwifery Council (NMC) has standards of competence that have to be met by applicants to different parts of the nursing and midwifery register. These standards are what the NMC deems necessary for the delivery of safe, effective nursing and midwifery practice. As well as specific competencies, the NMC identifies specific skills that nursing students must have at various points of their training programme. These Essential Skills Clusters (ESCs) are essential abilities that students need to attain in order to practise to their full potential.

This book identifies some of the competencies and skills within the realm of clinical judgement and decision-making that student nurses need in order to be entered onto the NMC register. These competencies and ESCs are presented at the start of each chapter so that it is clear which of them the chapter addresses. All of the competencies and ESCs in this book relate to the *generic standards* that all nursing students must achieve. This book includes the latest taken from the *Standards for pre-registration nursing education* (NMC, 2010).

Activities

At various stages within each chapter there are points at which you can break to undertake activities, and these are an important element of your understanding of the content of each chapter. You are encouraged, where appropriate, to reflect on your practice and consider how the things you have learnt from working with patients might inform your understanding of clinical judgement and decision-making. Other activities will require you to take time away from the book to find out new information that will add to your understanding of the topic under discussion. Some activities challenge you to apply your learning to a question or scenario to help you reflect on issues and practice in more depth. A few activities require you to make observations during your day-to-day life or in the clinical setting. All these activities are designed to increase your understanding of the topics under discussion and how they reflect on nursing practice.

Where appropriate, there are suggested or potential answers to activities at the end of the chapter. It is recommended that you try where possible to engage with the activities in order to increase your understanding of the realities of clinical judgement and decision-making.

A glossary explaining some of the more technical terms can be found at the back of the book. Terms included in the glossary will be in bold type the first time they appear.

Chapter 1
What is clinical judgement and decision-making in nursing?

NMC Standards for Pre-registration Nursing Education

This chapter will address the following competencies:

Domain 1: Professional values

5. All nurses must fully understand the nurse's various roles, responsibilities and functions, and adapt their practice to meet the changing needs of people, groups, communities and populations.

Domain 3: Nursing practice and decision-making

1. All nurses must use up-to-date knowledge and evidence to assess, plan, deliver and evaluate care, communicate findings, influence change and promote health and best practice. They must make person-centred, evidence-based judgements and decisions, in partnership with others involved in the care process, to ensure high quality care. They must be able to recognise when the complexity of clinical decisions requires specialist knowledge and expertise, and consult or refer accordingly.

Chapter aims

By the end of this chapter, you should be able to:

*   define clinical judgement and decision-making in nursing;
*   relate intuition, reflection and critical thinking to clinical judgement;
*   describe judgement and decision-making in planned, unplanned and emergency care;
*   relate concepts of human beings, environment, health and nursing to decision-making;
*   describe four criteria to review decision-making: practicality, logic, relevance and rigour;
*   apply ten perceptions of clinical decision-making to a patient's case study.

Introduction

The purpose of this chapter is to explain what **clinical judgement** and **clinical decision-making** in **nursing** mean, and stimulate your interest in reading the remainder of the book. It gives you a taste of what is to come in the way it uses case studies to help bring the subject to life and activities to help you to relate theory to your own experience and clinical practice. Collectively, the case studies used in this book are applicable to the full range of pre-registration nursing pathways (adult, child, mental health and learning disabilities). Case studies are a good way to explore decision-making, as the following case study illustrates.

Case study: Car crash

Roger, aged 44, is about to go and pick up his son from university for the Christmas vacation. It is a cold day and the sky is overcast, but it is dry. Roger is aware there have been reports of snow in other parts of England and Wales, expected to move his way by nightfall. He decides to set off early enough to complete the 220-mile return journey before it gets dark. Twenty minutes into the journey it begins to snow heavily; gritting lorries are working to prevent it from settling on the motorway, but two lanes are already covered in 5 cm of snow. Roger has experience of driving in these conditions, so although he is surprised by it coming so early, he chooses to carry on. He sees a 50 mph speed restriction is enforced and checks how fast he is going (45 mph). He is following a lorry. He cannot see that further up the road a car has skidded into the crash barrier. The back of the lorry is thick with dirt and snow, and Roger is unable to see that its brake lights are on. He suddenly realises he is going to smash into the lorry.

Roger takes his foot off the accelerator and changes to a lower gear, but the wheels do not grip and he does not slow down enough. He frantically 'pumps' the foot brake to try to slow down without skidding, but it is too late. He is half a second away from driving into the back of the lorry. In desperation he steers the car away and tries to thread his way through traffic in the inner lane but the steering is not very responsive in such slippery conditions. Roger collides with one car and is hit by another, all the airbags are deployed, and front and rear windscreens are broken by the force of impact. He manages to stop the car on the hard shoulder. The car is a write-off (damaged beyond economical repair), and Roger is badly shaken up. The car that was behind him ploughs into the back of the lorry, and the driver is treated for neck injuries. A police investigation rules that no one can be held responsible for what happened.

There were no fatalities in the case study, but road traffic accidents in England and Wales claimed 1645 lives (1228 males, 417 females) in 2015 (ONS, 2016a). It is possible that Roger escaped serious injury by avoiding contact with both the lorry in front of him and the car behind him.

Although the police ruled out prosecuting anyone for causing the accident by dangerous driving, it is important to look at how it might have been prevented to increase road safety. Activity 1.1 asks you some questions to explore this further.

Activity 1.1   *Decision-making*

The questions in this activity are intended to help you to uncover different aspects of decision-making with reference to the case study:

1. What were the different decisions that Roger made in the case study?
2. What sources of information did Roger use to base his decisions on?
3. In what way was Roger's driving style adapted to the road conditions?
4. What could Roger have done differently to avoid having an accident?
5. What might the lorry driver have done to help prevent the accident?
6. Do you think the trip itself was really necessary or not? Why?
7. How successful were the outcomes of Roger's decision-making?
8. In what way might Roger be held accountable for what happened?

Some possible answers can be found at the end of the chapter.

The case study and Activity 1.1 help us to piece together key characteristics of decision-making.

- Decision-making applies judgement regarding our reasons for doing or not doing things.
- We use different information sources to support our judgement and decision-making.
- It involves choices about what, when, where, why and how we do things, and with or for whom.
- Evaluating decision-making involves assessing the choices made and their effectiveness.
- Decisions can be planned, unplanned or an urgent reaction to an emergency situation.
- We are always making different types of decisions, often without realising that we are.
- Freedom to make decisions is balanced by **accountability** in having to answer for them.

The Transforming Nursing Practice series of books is well suited to exploring decision-making because they encourage learning through participation, thereby linking theory to practice. Similarly, clinical decision-making is the means by which we relate **nursing theory** and research to practice in carrying out nursing care for our patients.

This chapter begins by clarifying what we mean by clinical judgement and decision-making in nursing. We will briefly look at the development of nursing as a profession and how this impacts on our clinical decision-making. The structure of the book is then explained with reference to a research study on nursing students' development of clinical decision-making skills (Standing, 2005, 2007, 2010a), followed by a summary. More case studies and learning activities are used to engage you in the process.

What is clinical judgement and decision-making?

Nursing, like driving a car, involves carefully planned decisions (care plans), reacting to changing circumstances with unplanned decision-making (a patient looks upset so you check out why) and life-saving decisions in emergency situations (patient is choking so clear airway). This is why clinical judgement and decision-making have been acknowledged as key processes in nursing. For example, the Royal College of Nursing (RCN) defines nursing as:

the use of clinical judgement in the provision of care to enable people to improve, maintain, or recover health, to cope with health problems, and to achieve the best possible quality of life, whatever their disease or disability, until death.
(RCN, 2014a, p3)

This indicates that a nurse's ability to promote health, prevent illness, relieve suffering and give patients high quality care is dependent on applying effective clinical judgement. For the purposes of this book clinical judgement is defined as:

informed opinion (using intuition, reflection and critical thinking) that relates observation and assessment of patients to identifying and evaluating alternative nursing options.

In other words, clinical judgement involves assessing the potential consequences (risks and benefits) of possible alternative actions before committing oneself one way or the other (decision-making). For example, a nurse sees a boy who is recovering from surgery leaning out of bed trying to reach his glasses, which have fallen on the floor. The nurse is worried that he might open his wound or fall out of bed, so she quickly picks up the glasses (intuition). The nurse thought that if she did nothing, there was a risk the boy would be injured (reflection). On balance, she regarded the potential benefits of her actions – promoting wound healing and preventing painful injury – outweighed the potential risks – the boy might be annoyed that he was prevented from picking up the glasses for himself (critical thinking).

Decision-making links judgement to practice by acting on it in choosing from the available options (nurse picks up glasses in the example above). We are also accountable for the quality, safety and effectiveness of our clinical decision-making, as follows:

The nurse is a safe, caring and competent decision maker willing to accept personal and professional accountability for his/her actions and continuous learning. The nurse practises within a statutory framework and code of ethics delivering nursing practice (care) that is appropriately based on research, evidence and critical thinking that effectively responds to the needs of individual clients (patients) and diverse populations.
(Gonzalez and Wagenaar, 2003, cited in NMC, 2010, p11)

Nurses' clinical judgement and decision-making are informed by evidence ranging from observations of patients to research studies. They are also responsive to and aided by patients' preferences, healthcare colleagues' opinions and systems/policies/procedures that ensure care is of a professional standard. Figure 1.1 shows how different aspects of clinical judgement inform decision-making according to the time available to address health problems.

Figure 1.1 indicates that where there is no time to make decisions, such as in emergency situations (e.g. in the case study when Roger avoided the lorry), we rely more on intuitive judgement. Where there is more time to make decisions, our judgement needs to be informed by a critical review of relevant evidence (e.g. road safety information and training by RoSPA – Royal Society for the Prevention of Accidents). In between these contrasting approaches we use reflective,

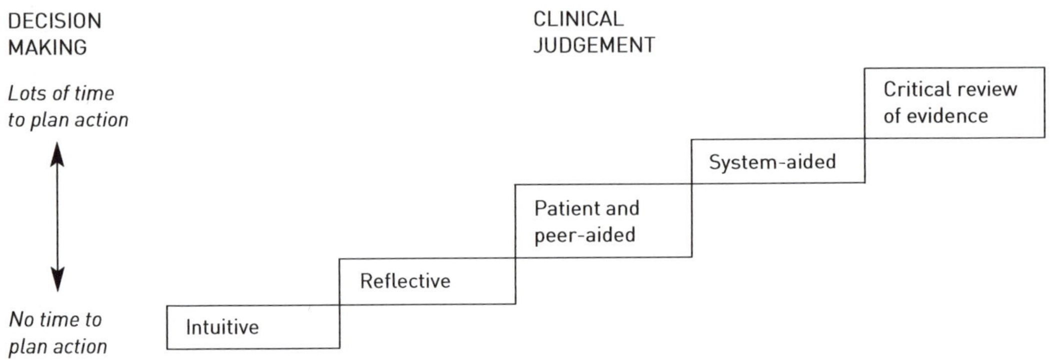

DECISION
MAKING

CLINICAL
JUDGEMENT

*Lots of time
to plan action*

*No time to
plan action*

	Critical review of evidence
	System-aided
	Patient and peer-aided
	Reflective
Intuitive	

Figure 1.1: Cognitive continuum matching clinical judgement to time for decision-making

Source: Adapted from Standing, 2005, 2008, 2010b

patient/peer-aided and system-aided clinical judgement according to the nature of the problem, relevant evidence and time available to take action. In effect, we use a **cognitive continuum** of judgement ranging from intuitive hunches to critical analysis that is tailored to the constantly changing nature of the clinical demands and health problems that we deal with (Hammond, 1996; Standing, 2010b).

The benefit of intuition is that it is quick and responsive to the immediate situation facing you. Its drawback is that human perception and judgement are prone to error and bias. The benefit of analysis is that relevant research evidence is used to inform action and minimise errors of judgement. Its drawbacks are that it is slow and that research may not have answers to all the issues in local contexts that make each decision unique. This book will help you to develop clinical judgement across the cognitive continuum so that your decisions will be responsive to individual needs and local contexts while being informed by relevant research and other evidence. Clinical decision-making converts clinical judgement into nursing interventions to address health problems, and for the purposes of this book it is defined as follows:

> *Clinical decision-making applies clinical judgement to select the best possible evidence-based option to control risks and address patients' needs in high quality care for which you are accountable.*

Activity 1.2 gives you a chance to clarify your understanding of the terminology.

Activity 1.2   *Reflection*

Think about what has been said in this section and answer the following questions as best you can.

1. What are the similarities and differences between clinical judgement and decision-making?
2. What are the benefits of good clinical judgement and decision-making skills in nursing?
3. How would you describe critical thinking skills, and why are they so important in nursing?

Some possible answers can be found at the end of the chapter.

Development of nursing, key concepts and clinical decision-making

Developing our decision-making ability is not a substitute for learning about the wide range of knowledge, skills and attitudes needed in nursing. With this in mind, key concepts of humans, environment, health and nursing (Fawcett and DeSanto-Madeya, 2012) are adapted to structure Table 1.1, which summarises over 150 years of professional development and its impact on our roles, clinical judgement and decision-making.

The idea of condensing and presenting you with a 'potted history' of nursing in Table 1.1 is not to press a panic button about names, dates and theories that you might be unfamiliar with – you are not expected to memorise it. It is something that offers a coherent overview of the key concepts and principles of nursing, the diverse scope of our roles as nurses, and the range of information sources and processes used in our clinical judgement and decision-making.

Human being

You have no doubt heard of the terms **person-centred**, client-centred and **patient-centred care**, but are you sure what they mean? The concept 'human being' (Table 1.1) offers a way to make sense of these 'buzz words'. For example, our uniqueness as individuals is both genetically and environmentally determined, and this will manifest itself in our physical and psychological characteristics, cultural values, variations in social behaviour, self-care ability and response to nursing care. Despite our differences we are all entitled to have our human rights protected during healthcare. This is explored in more depth in Chapter 2 (Collaborative clinical decision-making) and Chapter 9 (Ethical sensitivity in decision-making).

Environment and health

The concepts of environment and health are closely intertwined. Obvious examples include extreme variations in temperature, flooding, earthquakes and destructive winds, which claim many lives every year. Staying healthy therefore entails avoiding dangerous situations (e.g. not driving in the snow) and unhealthy habits (e.g. not smoking). Some threats are less visible, such as viruses, which are particularly dangerous to the most vulnerable. Preventative medicine helps to minimise these risks; for example, young children are vaccinated against mumps, measles and rubella (MMR), and older adults are vaccinated against influenza. Environments we expect to be safe, such as the home, may not always be so. If children are abused by parents, they need to be removed to a place of safety before it is too late. Sometimes work environments are unsafe. On 24 April 2013 a nine-storey clothing factory in Bangladesh collapsed, killing 1129 factory workers. The factory owners and local mayor (who allowed the unsafe structure to be built) were arrested and charged with manslaughter. We are all accountable if our actions endanger others. For some people, surviving in hostile environments is an everyday reality and duty, and the health of those who do survive can be affected for the rest of their lives, as the next case study illustrates.

Concepts	Meanings of, interaction between, and relevance of concepts
Human being	• Shaped by nature (genetically predetermined traits) and nurture (constant interaction physically, psychologically and socially with the environment). Range of biological, psychological, social, philosophical and spiritual needs. • Developmental milestones during lifespan: from birth – dependent child, adolescent, creative independent adult, less independent old age – to death. • Basic human rights to life, self-determination, freedom from oppression. • Self-care ability: resist infection, recover from injury/illness, adapt to disability.
Environment	• Physical: air, food, water, warmth, shelter, natural resources to support life. • Social: family, culture, politics/economics/law, education, religion, technology (Leininger, 1985).
Health	• *Physical, mental and social wellbeing and not merely the absence of disease or infirmity* (WHO, 1948); product of interaction between human beings and environment to address their needs (health) or not to (ill health); variations between cultures in how health and ill health are interpreted.
Nursing (role and clinical decision-making)	• Human advocacy: enable and empower people to adopt healthy lifestyle, prevent ill health, get relief from suffering, recover from illness or injury, adapt to disability and have a peaceful death (RCN, 2014a). • Nursing theories' view of role: keep environment clean to promote healing (Nightingale, 1860); help people to address bio-psycho-social-spiritual needs or activities of living (Henderson, 1966; Roper et al., 2000); use interpersonal relationships, therapeutic communication and cultural sensitivity in enabling people to cope with stress, enhance mental health and find meaning in their lives (Peplau, 1952; Leininger, 1985; Parse, 1992); encourage holistic (bio-psycho-social) self-care or adaptation by tailoring interventions according to a person's level of dependence or independence (Orem, 1980; Roy, 1980); apply principles of human caring to achieve all of the above (Watson, 1988). • Clinical decision-making in nursing is informed by: systematic problem solving (Yura and Walsh, 1973); reflective practice (Schön, 1983); expert intuitive judgement (Benner, 1984); and accessing, evaluating and applying research in evidence-based practice (Cullum et al., 2007; Ellis, 2016).

Table 1.1: Key concepts in nursing: relevance to nurses' role and decision-making

> ### Case study: The retired explosives expert (i)
>
> *William is 71 years old. He joined the British Army when he was 18, and at 21 he was a tank commander; this was when he first noticed hearing problems. After undergoing commando and paratrooper training he became an explosives expert – laying bombs to kill enemy troops during jungle warfare in Borneo, and detecting and defusing bombs intended to kill his colleagues in Northern Ireland. William left the army as a sergeant major at the age of 33. Apart from sustaining marked hearing loss, his right leg and his arms were scarred, and small fragments of shrapnel remained embedded beneath his skin. He was also psychologically affected by the loss of several colleagues killed in action. He became an explosives contractor, extracting building materials from quarries across Africa. He retired at the age of 65 and returned to England with his wife and their two children. Over the years William has spent thousands of pounds on hearing aids.*

William's hearing problems might have been prevented if he had been given protective ear muffs when firing his tank's big gun and when detonating bombs. Nowadays soldiers undertaking similar duties are issued with hearing protectors. We will revisit William's case study when exploring decision-making criteria in nursing.

Nursing

The concept of nursing in Table 1.1 reminds us that our first duty is to champion the health and wellbeing of our patients. The overview of theories conveys the breadth and depth of **holistic** (bio-psycho-socio-spiritual) knowledge associated with nursing, applicable to all the pathways. Collectively, the theories support patient-centred, interpersonally skilled, holistic, systematic, critical, reflective, health-promoting, evidence-based, culturally sensitive and caring nursing. These attributes are also found in the *Standards for pre-registration nursing education* (NMC, 2010).

According to Snyder (1995), *The theoretical or conceptual model used by a nurse provides the basis for making complex decisions that are crucial in the delivery of good nursing care* (p33). However, when the RCN surveyed nurses about their understanding of nursing (in compiling a definition), they discovered that many nurses found it hard to describe their knowledge or skills. Similarly, Clark (2006) reported that nurses often *find it difficult to put into words the concept of nursing that they hold inside their heads* (p33). For theory to enhance practice it must be accessible, understandable, relevant and applicable. If the language used to explain ideas is complicated or confusing, then even if it contains useful information, it will not be understood. A **theory–practice gap** occurs where the formal learning of **espoused theories** in universities is in conflict with informal, work-based **theories-in-use** in professional practice (Argyris and Schön, 1974). As stated in the introduction, clinical decision-making involves theory applied to practice, and it is important that we are able to explain reasons for nursing actions. If we are unable to, how can we enable patients to give informed consent to treatment and care?

The final subsection of 'nursing' in Table 1.1 describes the emergence of a range of clinical decision-making approaches associated with different aspects of clinical judgement and levels of **critical thinking** (see also Figure 1.1). Intuitive judgement is valuable when decisions have to be made quickly, but as it tends to function at a subconscious level, it is often difficult to clearly articulate reasons for decisions. Critical review and application of research-based evidence is valuable when there is time to plan care thoroughly, and as it is a conscious process of judgement and decision-making, it is open to scrutiny by others. This enables the communication of nursing knowledge and skills, and greater public accountability for decision-making, which are important because:

- nurses need to consult, negotiate, discuss and explain the reasons for their proposed practical care to patients, families, other nurses and members of the healthcare team;
- nurses need to keep clear written records as evidence of the care they have provided;
- each nurse is accountable for the quality of care (its safety and effectiveness) that they give to patients, and must be able to justify and defend their actions if challenged to do so.

Figure 1.2 links developments in nursing to four vital criteria of safe and effective clinical judgement/decision-making: practicality, logic, relevance and rigour (Standing and Standing, 2010).

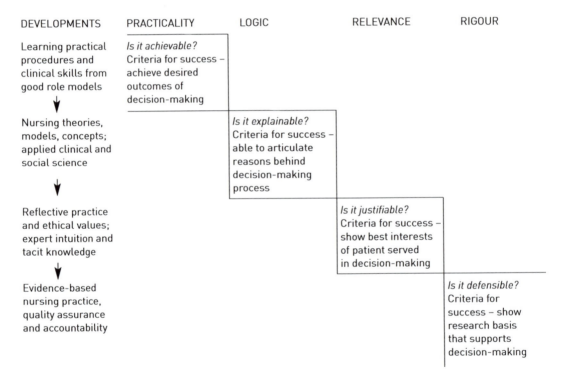

Figure 1.2: Developments in nursing in relation to four vital decision-making criteria

In order to see how the criteria of practicality, logic, relevance and rigour are applied in reviewing the quality of nurses' clinical decision-making, we will revisit the case study about William.

Case study: The retired explosives expert (ii)

William has medication to control high blood pressure, and he attends the health centre to have his blood pressure monitored. While having this done he mentions to Joan (the practice nurse) that his consultant audiologist has told him his hearing has deteriorated and he needs new hearing aids in both ears. William says it is going to 'cost him a fortune' and that his only income is his state pension. Joan asks why he does not have an army pension, and William explains that after he left the army he found out that if he had stayed for two more weeks he would have qualified for an army pension reflecting his years served, as well as the state pension when he turned 65. When Joan has some free time she uses the internet to research William's possible entitlement to financial help and discovers that he might be eligible for a War Disablement Pension. William 'does not get on with computers' so she prints off the application forms for him. Months later William has a medical assessment by an army doctor who confirms he is eligible for a War Disablement Pension, payable from the date of the assessment. This helps to offset the cost of his new hearing aids.

Joan's actions are consistent with the two NMC Standards and competencies identified at the beginning of this chapter. Rather than just sticking to the task of recording blood pressure, Joan was also responsive to William's other concerns. In doing so she showed how nurses *adapt their practice to meet the changing needs of people* and *make person-centred, evidence-based judgements and decisions*. We can now review Joan's action in relation to the four decision-making criteria identified earlier.

1. *Practicality*: Is it achievable? Yes: there was a good outcome as William was successful in getting a War Disablement Pension. If Joan had not taken the initiative, he would not have known about his entitlement. As William did not use computers it was vital that Joan printed the forms for him.
2. *Logic*: Is it explainable? Yes: Joan knew that exposure to loud noises causes hearing loss. William had reported a history of this in the army. She found information and entitlement criteria about the War Disablement Pension from the Service Personnel and Veterans Agency (SPVA).
3. *Relevance*: Is it justifiable? Yes: William just missed out on getting an army pension and was unaware that he could have applied for the War Disablement Pension years before. Enabling William to be compensated for his disability helps to pay for hearing aids and ease his financial worries.
4. *Rigour*: Is it defensible? Yes: Joan adopted a questioning approach to probe William's concerns about the cost of hearing aids. She demonstrated evidence-based decision-making in facilitating his application to get help. His medical history and examination provided corroborating evidence.

We can see that Joan successfully addressed the decision-making criteria of practicality, logic, relevance and rigour. In doing so she integrated and applied knowledge, skills, attitudes and values associated with the development of nursing shown in Table 1.1 and Figure 1.2 (practical procedures, nursing theory, reflective practice and **evidence-based practice**). The unique structure of this book will help you to develop these skills and we will revisit the decision-making criteria in Chapter 12 so you can evaluate your progress.

The book's unique structure: ten perceptions of clinical decision-making

The research study

The book's structure is shaped by a unique research study (using **hermeneutic phenomenology**) exploring nursing students' experiences of clinical decision-making on a four-year developmental journey in becoming and practising as registered nurses (Standing, 2005, 2009).

Twenty students kept reflective journals of their experiences in acquiring and applying clinical decision-making skills throughout the pre-registration programme and first year as staff nurses (adult/mental health/child) between 2000 and 2004 (there was no learning disability pathway at the institution in question). This was supplemented by four tape-recorded in-depth interviews with each student (at 3–5, 18–20, 32–34 and 42–48 months). The interviews helped students to recall and discuss critical incidents they had experienced and to clarify their personal conceptions (understanding) of nursing, and their perceptions of clinical decision-making skills. A total of 250,000 words of interview transcripts were generated, and these were thematically analysed, revealing ten conceptions of nursing and ten perceptions of clinical decision-making. The themes were checked with the students, and developed and refined as necessary to accurately reflect their views, and to summarise their experiences.

A 'Matrix model' was created by cross-referencing nursing conceptions with perceptions of clinical decision-making (Standing, 2005, 2007, 2010a). It helps nurses to integrate key concepts, skills, attitudes and values with the clinical decision-making criteria in Table 1.1 and Figure 1.2. Table 1.2 lists the conceptions of nursing and perceptions of clinical decision-making. Each of the next ten chapters is dedicated to a detailed exploration of a different perception of decision-making which are reviewed by cross-referencing them with the ten conceptions of nursing.

The themes in Table 1.2 summarise students' personal, practical and theoretical understanding of clinical decision-making, and support the view that *Professional practice requires knowledge derived from research and theory, from professional practice, and from personal experience* (Higgs and Titchen, 2001, pp4–5). The themes complement the nursing theories referred to earlier and *Standards for pre-registration nursing education* (NMC, 2010). Collectively they represent a system of delivering high quality, compassionate nursing care as advocated by the Department of Health's policy document *Compassion in practice* (DH, 2012a).

Conceptions of nursing	Perceptions of clinical decision-making
Caring	Collaborative
Listening and being there	Observation
Practical procedures	Systematic
Knowledge and understanding	Standardised
Communicating	Prioritising
Patience	Experience and intuition
Teamwork	Reflective
Paperwork and electronic record	Ethical sensitivity
Empathising and non-judgemental	Accountability
Professional	Confidence

Table 1.2: Nurses' understanding of nursing and clinical decision-making skills

Applying ten perceptions of decision-making

We will look at each perception of decision-making in detail in Chapters 2–11, but first we will look at a case study in which all ten perceptions are applied, to give you a flavour of the book as a whole. The case study shows that if a nursing student is observant, they can make a real and positive difference to a vulnerable person's life and complement the role of an experienced nurse and healthcare team.

Case study: Frightened to use the lift

Pearl is a second-year nursing student on placement in a community health centre. She goes with Shirley, a district nurse, to take a blood sample from Maude, aged 73, who is unable to get out much due to her arthritis. Maude's mobility is also hampered because she lives on the eighteenth floor of a high-rise block of flats (owned by the local council). While Shirley is attending to Maude, Pearl talks to her daughter Beth, aged 32, who has Down's syndrome (a genetic abnormality that is associated with intellectual disability and unusual appearance – flat face, slanting eyes, small mouth, and sometimes protruding tongue and fingers with webbed skin). Beth asks Pearl if she would like a cup of tea, adding that the people in the church hall, where she volunteers, always say she makes a lovely cup of tea. Pearl, seeing that Beth's hands are blistered, says, 'Not at the moment, thank you' and asks, 'What happened to your hands?' Beth's demeanour changes from cheerful to serious and sad. She tells Pearl that since she has been doing all the shopping, a nasty

(Continued)

continued . . .

family on the seventh floor calls her horrible names if they see her in the lift. She has asked them to stop, but they just do it more. So, for the last six months Beth has only used the lift between the eighth and eighteenth floors. She walks up and down seven flights of stairs between the ground floor and the eighth floor to avoid seeing the 'nasty' family and has blisters from pulling the fully laden trolley up the stairs. Pearl says she is sorry to hear that she is being bullied and asks if Beth has told her mum about what has happened. Beth says she hasn't because it is her job to look after her mum now.

Pearl reports this to Shirley, who praises Beth for doing such a great job of looking after her mum but adds that she must also look after herself. Keeping the bullying a secret will not make it stop, and if she falls down the stairs, nobody will know she is there. They agree a plan for Shirley to inform the GP, council, social services and police so that the offending family are made to stop bullying Beth. Although Maude loves the view from her flat, she agrees that it might also be time to ask the council for more suitable accommodation nearer the ground. In the meantime, Beth will arrange to go shopping with a friendly neighbour so that she feels safe using the lift all the way from the ground to the eighteenth floor. Beth asks Pearl how to send texts on the mobile phone her mum ordered for her, and Pearl shows her this and also how to store numbers. Beth practises texting and storing numbers with Pearl's help and is happy that she can now text her friends. Shirley tells Pearl that she did a really good job in finding out about Beth being bullied.

The case study brings into perspective the key concepts outlined in Table 1.1. Beth's rights as a human being had been violated just because she looked different from other people. Problems getting in and out of the block of flats highlight the way in which the physical and social environment can affect someone's health and wellbeing (too frightened to use the lift). With regard to her nursing skills, Pearl was caring, attentive and empathising, and she communicated with Beth in a way she felt comfortable with. She applied technical skills in showing Beth how to send texts on her mobile phone and demonstrated teamwork skills by informing Shirley about the bullying. The range of clinical decision-making used by Shirley, Pearl and other agencies is summarised in Table 1.3. The main thrust of short-term decision-making was focused on safeguarding Beth by implementing legal sanctions to stop the offenders if necessary, and ensuring that Beth feels safe when she goes out shopping. In the longer term, it is likely that Maude and Beth will be rehoused.

Applying the ten perceptions to the case study reveals a wide range of knowledge, skills and values needed by adult, mental health, child and learning disability nurses in their clinical judgement and decision-making. In reality many of these skills are used simultaneously, but in order to learn more about them we will explore them one at a time in Chapters 2–11.

The importance of the decisions taken to safeguard and protect Beth in this case study is graphically illustrated in Chapter 2 when a mother and daughter with intellectual disabilities are not given the support they deserve.

Perceptions of decision-making	Examples of decision-making in the case study
Collaborative	Telling GP/council housing officer/social services/police that Beth is being bullied.
Observation	Noticing Beth's hands were blistered and that it seemed to be worrying her.
Systematic	Authorities investigate – tell bullies to stop or face eviction and prosecution.
Standardised	Discrimination illegal (Equality Act 2010) and breaches tenancy agreement.
Prioritising	Stopping the bullying for Beth to use lift safely; reviewing housing options.
Experience and intuition	Sensing Beth is unhappy; identifying the problem by enabling her to talk about it.
Reflective	Asking Beth to go out with a buddy she feels safe with; her neighbour agrees.
Ethical sensitivity	Respecting Beth's right to come and go in the lift without fear of intimidation.
Accountability	Professional obligation to safeguard a vulnerable adult if abuse suspected.
Confidence	Enabling Beth to send/read texts and store numbers on her mobile phone.

Table 1.3: Applying ten perceptions of decision-making to the case study

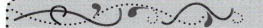

Chapter summary

This chapter introduced you to clinical judgement and decision-making for nursing students. We began by clarifying what the terms meant and their similarities and differences. We noted that there is a range of clinical judgement from intuitive (with less critical thinking) to critical review of evidence (with more critical thinking), and that these were related to fast, unplanned decision-making and slow, well-planned decision-making, respectively. We noted that intuition is responsive to the local context but prone to human error, while critical analysis of research evidence is more rigorous but may not have all the answers needed to manage situations. We had a brief overview of the historical development of

(Continued)

continued . . .

nursing as a profession regarding key concepts – human being, environment, health and nursing. We saw how this can help us understand and explain nursing knowledge, skills, attitudes and values – for example, what 'patient-centred' means. We skipped through a variety of nursing theories supporting a holistic understanding of people. We looked at various approaches to clinical decision-making in nursing, how each one has particular strengths and how combining them all seems sensible, and we looked at vital criteria – practicality, logic, relevance and rigour – to quality-assure decision-making. A research study was described that followed a group of students through the nursing programme and first year as staff nurses to explore how they identified, developed and applied clinical decision-making skills. Ten wide-ranging perceptions of decision-making were identified from the research, which will be used as the basis for the next ten chapters in this book. They will be cross-referenced to conceptions of nursing identified in the research study (Standing, 2005, 2007, 2010a) to integrate professional values and compassionate care within nurses' clinical decision-making. The final case study (pages 15–16) showed how all ten perceptions of decision-making were used in caring for a vulnerable adult who had been victimised. It also enabled us to see how theoretical concepts (human being, environment, health and nursing) are applied in compassionate evidence-based practice. In Chapter 4 of this book we will see how these key concepts inform an 'activities of living' model (Roper et al., 2000) when nursing someone with a long-term medical condition. Each remaining chapter will build on this one in developing your knowledge, skills, attitudes and values in clinical judgement and decision-making. I hope this chapter has whetted your appetite.

Activities: brief outline answers

Activity 1.1: Decision-making (page 6)

You may have included the following points.

1. What were the different decisions that Roger made in the case study? To collect son from university; timing of trip; continuing despite snow; avoiding lorry.
2. What sources of information did Roger use to base his decisions on? Looked at sky; heard weather forecast; observing road conditions; judgements of speed and distance.
3. In what way was Roger's driving style adapted to the road conditions? Kept within speed restriction; tried to slow down with gears to avoid skidding.
4. What could Roger have done differently to avoid having an accident? Not gone; researched weather forecast more thoroughly; turned back when it snowed; kept longer distance from lorry in front; changed lane before so he was not behind lorry and could see road ahead more clearly.
5. What might the lorry driver have done to help prevent the accident? Cleaned back of lorry to make brake lights visible; stayed on the inner lane.
6. Do you think the trip itself was really necessary or not? Why? With hindsight, risks outweighed benefits given surprising early snowfall.
7. How successful were the outcomes of Roger's decision-making? Unsuccessful: failed to pick up son; car was a write-off; hit/got hit by other cars. Successful: avoided more serious injury by avoiding driving into the back of the lorry.
8. In what way might Roger be held accountable for what happened? Police checking if anyone was to blame – but concluding 'no'; telling son he cannot make it; may lose no claims bonus; vehicle he hit may claim off his insurance.

Activity 1.2: Reflection (page 8)

You may have included the following points.

1. *Similarities* – both are used to define nursing; apply critical thinking; consider alternative options; apply theory to practice. *Differences* – one assesses options, the other chooses and implements one of the options.
2. *Benefits* – high quality, evidence-based nursing that addresses patients' healthcare needs.
3. *Description* – questioning assumptions of self and others, addressing gaps in knowledge needed to achieve aims, challenging illogical beliefs, evaluating adequacy of research evidence, presenting a logical, evidence-based argument and defending it when challenged. *Importance* – without it, you cannot achieve the above benefits; registered nurses are accountable and have to justify their actions when challenged.

Further reading

Ellis, P (2016) *Evidence-based practice in nursing* (3rd edn). London: Sage/Learning Matters.

A good introduction to a wide range of evidence used to inform clinical judgement and decisions.

Hall, C and Ritchie, D (2013) *What is nursing?* (3rd edn). London: Sage/Learning Matters.

Helpful overview of the theory and practice of nursing.

Holland, K and Roberts, D (2013) *Nursing: decision-making skills for practice.* Oxford: Oxford University Press.

Alternative introduction to decision-making to help students to prepare for practice in different pathways.

McKenna, H, Pajnkihar, M and Murphy, F (2014) *Fundamentals of nursing models, theories and practice* (2nd edn). Oxford: Wiley/Blackwell.

A useful exploration of nursing models and theories, which raises interesting questions about whether and how they are used in practice.

Useful websites

www.mencap.org.uk

Website of the learning disabilities charity. Very informative and supportive with lots of interesting video clips.

www.nursing-theory.org

This website has helpful summaries of the nursing theories/models referred to in Chapter 1 plus many more, and it contains useful links to more detailed information if desired.

www.rospa.com/road-safety

Website of the Royal Society for the Prevention of Accidents charity which is dedicated to improving standards of driving/riding and behaviour of drivers/riders, e.g. hazard perception and fitness to drive.

Chapter 2
Collaborative clinical decision-making

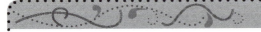

continued . . .

6. People can trust the newly registered graduate nurse to engage therapeutically and actively listen to their needs and concerns, responding using skills that are helpful, providing information that is clear, accurate, meaningful and free from jargon.

Cluster: Organisational aspects of care

11. People can trust the newly registered graduate nurse to safeguard children and adults from vulnerable situations and support and protect them from harm.

12. People can trust the newly registered graduate nurse to respond to their feedback and a wide range of other sources to learn, develop and improve services.

Chapter aims

By the end of this chapter, you should be able to:

- explain what collaborative clinical decision-making means;
- give examples of collaborative decision-making with patients;
- describe collaborative decision-making within the healthcare team;
- understand your role in collaborating with healthcare team members;
- appreciate that collaboration is vital for integrated patient-centred care.

Introduction

This chapter and the next nine chapters of the book each explore a different clinical decision-making theme, identified when researching nursing students' experience and perceptions of their developmental journey in becoming (and practising as) registered nurses (Standing, 2005, 2007, 2010a). Of the ten themes identified in the research we begin with **collaborative decision-making**.

1. There was more agreement about the importance of collaborative decision-making by nurses in the research study than about any of the other themes they identified.
2. Collaboration underpins the '6Cs' of care, compassion, competence, communication, courage and commitment that are essential in order to give *high quality, compassionate care and to achieve excellent health and wellbeing outcomes* (DH, 2012a, p28).
3. This and subsequent chapters will help you to participate in a collaborative way by testing out ideas presented and relating them to your experience.

This suggests that collaboration is central not only to nursing practice and management but also to nursing research and education. Collaborative decision-making, therefore, seems a logical starting point on our journey in exploring together nurses' clinical decision-making skills.

The chapter begins by asking 'What is collaborative decision-making?' and looking at the similarities and differences between collaboration, co-operation, consultation, negotiation and collusion. These issues are then related to our professional context by asking, 'What is collaborative clinical decision-making in nursing?' The rest of the chapter is dedicated to applying collaborative clinical decision-making in nursing: (i) when working in partnership with patients and families; (ii) when working in partnership with health and social care professionals and other agencies; and (iii) when integrating working with patients/families and various health and social care workers in order to give high quality care. Practical examples and case studies illustrate applications of collaborative decision-making in different clinical contexts. Various activities encourage you to relate chapter contents to your own personal and clinical experience. Finally, the strengths and weaknesses of collaborative clinical decision-making are summarised.

What is collaborative decision-making?

Collaborative decisions are joint decisions between two or more people for the purpose of achieving an agreed aim. For example, in the build up to the United Kingdom's (UK) referendum on European Union (EU) membership in 2016, the official policy of all of the political parties who had experience in national government was for the UK to remain in the EU. So, despite their political differences they agreed to collaborate in campaigning for a remain vote. However, they were unsuccessful as a majority (albeit slim) of UK citizens taking part in the referendum voted to leave. Collaboration does not therefore guarantee successful outcomes but the process itself is democratic and is made up of three interrelated elements:

- Consultation to communicate concerns and discuss how to resolve them.
- Negotiation to identify a plan which all parties can agree to and act upon.
- Co-operation to suspend potential differences and work together to achieve shared aims.

All three elements are needed in collaborative decision-making in trying to achieve desired outcomes. For example, enabling everyone to have their say is of limited use if their views are ignored when decisions are being made. Plans to tackle problems are limited if they are not implemented as agreed. A commitment to working together is limited if 'not rocking the boat' inhibits debate or cultivates begrudging compliance to the most dominant view. Hence, combining and balancing consultation, negotiation and co-operation are essential to enable democratic participation, power sharing, effective discussion, agreement and joint action in collaborative decision-making.

Activity 2.1   *Decision-making*

Describe your involvement in collaborative decisions outside nursing – for example, what to cook, what film to watch, where to go on holiday, when to go shopping. Identify what you had in common with those with whom you agreed decisions and the aims you think you shared. Reflect on how easy or difficult it was to agree what to do, what each person's contribution to the process was and how successful you think the outcome was for all those concerned.

- What are the key features of collaborative decision-making that your examples illustrate?

Some possible answers are included at the end of the chapter.

The word 'collaboration' can also have negative associations. For example, a 'collaborator' during the Second World War was regarded as a traitor working with the enemy. Negative forms of collaboration involve collusion, subterfuge and sabotage where prevailing social, political or moral values are undermined by a shared, more secretive, alternative agenda. There is an inconsistency between what you say publicly you believe in and what you actually believe in and do 'behind the scenes'. Some examples are given below.

- The 'lid was lifted' on divisions within the Conservative majority government when a few high profile members broke ranks and joined the opposing side in campaigning to leave the EU.
- There were recriminations against Jeremy Corbyn, Labour leader, from his own members of parliament (MPs) for not doing more in their view to persuade the public to remain in the EU.
- If a nurse says nothing when a colleague forgets to wash their hands before attending to a patient's wound, then the nurse is colluding with the colleague in endangering the patient's health and safety (in this case health promotion values are undermined by a lack of assertiveness).

Activity 2.2 provides an opportunity for you to identify instances of collusion you might have come across.

Activity 2.2   *Reflection*

See if you can recall any examples of collusion from what you have observed or experienced. Briefly describe the circumstances and why you think those involved colluded with each other. These examples could be during your nursing programme, in clinical practice or in non-nursing contexts.

- How do your examples illustrate the characteristics of collusion described above?

Some possible answers are included at the end of the chapter.

We will look in more detail at the potential risks and consequences of collusion later in the chapter.

Positive forms of collaborative decision-making are democratic in nature and part of sustaining productive relationships in all aspects of human interaction (including healthcare), as illustrated in the case study below.

Case study: Give and take in relationships

At the beginning of their nursing programme, students were asked about their understanding and experience of decision-making. Jo talked about making joint decisions with her fiancé.

'Decision-making between the two of us is a 50–50 thing unless one has particularly strong views and the other hasn't. If we've both got strong views, then it's "telly off" and we have a debate about it. When

(Continued)

---

continued . . .

it comes to life decisions, he wants to join the fire brigade and I have been considering a nursing career in the army. We agreed to see whether he gets into the fire brigade. If he does, I can put off the army for a few years as I can be a nurse in the NHS or the army but he can only be a fireman in the fire brigade. It's very much "give and take"; I'll compromise or he'll compromise depending on what's more important and who can still be happy. I'll probably be happy working in an NHS A&E department or in an army field hospital in Afghanistan.'

The case study is an example of collaborative decision-making because it involves more than one person, the respective parties each make a distinct contribution and they work together to achieve a common aim. The aim in this instance is to enable the couple to maintain a sustainable partnership while realising their respective career ambitions, in a way that both are happy with. It involves listening to and respecting each person's opinions (consultation), flexibility to compromise where priorities may clash (negotiation) and goodwill in deferring some of one's own preferences, where necessary, to support others in achieving their goals (co-operation).

Activity 2.3   *Decision-making*

Identify a joint (collaborative) nursing decision that you were involved in or witnessed, and briefly describe who was involved, their respective contributions (including yours), the shared aim you were all hoping to achieve, the agreed decision, the action taken and the resulting outcome. Try to identify examples of:

- consultation – how each person's opinions were taken on board;
- negotiation – how agreement was reached about main priorities;
- co-operation – how behaviour was adjusted to achieve goals.

As this is to help you relate collaborative decision-making to your own experience, there is no outline answer provided.

Having identified and reflected on key aspects of collaborative decision-making, we can now look in more detail at how this relates to nurses' clinical decisions.

What is collaborative clinical decision-making in nursing?

The answer to this question incorporates what we mean by collaboration (discussed above), what we mean by clinical decision-making (defined in Chapter 1) and what we mean by nursing (discussed in Chapter 1). We will start by clarifying our understanding of nursing and then link this to collaborative clinical decision-making. For the purposes of this book, nursing is defined as follows.

> *Nursing promotes health and wellbeing, relief from suffering, recovery from illness or injury, adaptation to disability, and dignity when facing death, in patient-centred care applying bio-psycho-social-spiritual knowledge, skills and ethical values to ensure safe and effective clinical judgement and decision-making and high quality, evidence-based practice.*

We can relate this to the nurse–patient relationship between Joan and William who we met in Chapter 1. Joan promoted William's health by ensuring his blood pressure was not too high. She contributed to William's adaptation to his disability through evidence-based practice by researching financial support he might be entitled to. In doing so she was attentive to William's personal psychological and social/economic needs as well as his physical problems. Once she had given William the information and forms he needed to apply for a War Disablement Pension, it was his choice whether to fill them in and what to write down. The successful outcome was achieved by collaborative decision-making (consultation/negotiation/co-operation) between Joan, William, the army doctor and the pension provider.

The patient-centred focus of our nursing definition reinforces the importance of collaborating with patients and relatives. The broad scope of nursing activities (from promoting health to enabling a dignified death) also requires collaboration with other health professionals or agencies who have specialist skills to help identify or address patients' wide-ranging needs. The aim we all share is to promote or restore health and wellbeing and relieve suffering in giving high quality care that is relevant to patients' healthcare needs.

We cannot, therefore, give patient-centred nursing care without collaborating with patients and others. Being patient-centred involves: consulting with patients to identify their preferences and get feedback about their care; explaining options, giving information to help them decide if they consent to proposed treatments; negotiating and implementing action plans that are relevant and responsive to patients' unique needs; and co-operating with other healthcare professionals by working together as a team to achieve this. By putting together our understanding of nursing, decision-making and collaboration, we arrive at a definition for the purposes of this book.

> *Collaborative clinical decision-making in nursing involves consulting, negotiating and co-operating with patients, relatives, nurses, mentors, managers, health professionals and other relevant agencies to promote health and to inform the delivery of high quality, patient-centred care that is relevant to their specific needs.*

Each stage of good patient-centred nursing care requires collaborative decision-making with patients and families (sometimes referred to as service users and carers in public documents relating to healthcare). It often involves inter-professional or inter-agency collaboration through effective partnership and teamwork. Indeed, the readiness and ability to collaborate and work in partnership with patients, colleagues and other relevant parties is one of the defining characteristics of nurses according to the Royal College of Nursing:

> *A commitment to partnership: nurses work in partnership with patients, their relatives and other carers, and in collaboration with others as members of a multi-disciplinary team. Where appropriate they will lead the team, prescribing, delegating and supervising the work of others; at other times they will participate under the leadership of others. At all times, however, they remain personally and professionally accountable for their own decisions and actions.*
> (RCN, 2014a, p3)

Applying collaborative clinical decision-making in nursing

The application of collaborative clinical decision-making is an essential part of nurse–patient relationships and inter-professional teamwork in hospital and community health or social care settings. We start off by looking at collaborating with patients and families; this is followed by inter-professional collaboration and then how to integrate the two strands in collaborative healthcare.

Collaborating with patients and families

Collaborative clinical decision-making is dependent on establishing effective relationships with patients and families. However, learning how to communicate and consult with patients, in order to find out what their opinions and preferences are, can take a while to achieve, as illustrated in the following case study.

Case study: Conversations with patients

Connie is a nursing student nearing the end of her first year. She reflects on how she learnt to focus more on patients' needs during her conversations with them.

'I realise that I like talking to people. People that have been sitting in a hospital bed are bored and they often want to talk. There was an elderly lady who I took a "shine" to. I know you're not supposed to. I spent more time with her because she was more talkative than other people and I found it easy to think of things to say to her. Then I suddenly realised that she probably wasn't interested in what I was saying, and that it was she who really needed someone to talk to. I thought to myself "I will just let her do the talking", and since then I have been able to stop myself from "rambling away" with patients and been more attentive to what they might need.'

Connie became aware that her interest in talking to a patient reflected her personal needs rather than the patient's. This increased level of self-awareness enabled her to listen more and say less, in order to help patients talk about issues affecting them. In doing so, Connie indicated that she had translated her social conversation skills into purposeful, professional and patient-centred communication/interpersonal skills that increased her effectiveness in consulting with patients. In Activity 2.4 you are asked to think about your own experience of communicating with patients.

Activity 2.4   *Communication*

Think about and describe an experience in communicating with patients. Like Connie, you may find some patients easier and more interesting to talk to than others. Why do you think it is vital to have a good relationship and be skilled at consulting with *all* patients in eliciting their views?

Some possible answers are included at the end of the chapter.

Connie experienced a tension between using social conversation skills to establish relationships with patients and developing other therapeutic communication skills that focus more directly on addressing patients' concerns. Contact with patients provides continuous experiential learning opportunities to refine our communication skills while physically, emotionally and psychologically engaged in interpersonal therapeutic activities. In this way we learn to blend personal, practical and professional qualities in shaping our nursing identities and roles (Higgs and Titchen, 2001). We will be looking at this in more detail in Chapter 7, Experience and intuition in decision-making, and in Chapter 8, Reflective judgement and decision-making. Theoretical approaches can also help to inform nurses' understanding, development, application and validation of their communication and interpersonal skills (Bach and Grant, 2015). Without this ability to 'tune in' to what patients' healthcare concerns are, whether in hospital or at home, collaborative clinical decision-making with them is not really possible. The importance of understanding patients as individuals and collaborating with them throughout their care is highlighted in the 'Prioritise people' section of the Nursing and Midwifery Council's (NMC) code of professional standards of practice and behaviour, including the following:

2 Listen to people and respond to their preferences and concerns

To achieve this you must:

2.1 work in partnership with people to make sure you deliver care effectively

2.2 recognise and respect the contribution that people can make to their own health and wellbeing

2.3 encourage and empower people to share decisions about their treatment and care

2.4 respect the level to which people receiving care want to be involved in decisions about their own health, wellbeing and care
(NMC, 2015, pp4–5)

These requirements are also reflected in various *Standards* (and Essential Skills Clusters) *for pre-registration nursing education* (NMC, 2010), as revealed at the start of this chapter. Good listening, communication and interpersonal skills are therefore essential in order to work in partnership with the public and professional colleagues in prioritising (and collaborate in delivering) safe and effective patient/client/person-centred care.

Building on collaboration

Knowing that developing and maintaining a good nurse–patient relationship is an important factor in providing high quality care and enabling effective collaborative clinical decision-making does not guarantee it always happens in practice. Many areas of nursing are highly pressurised, and this can sometimes result in less consultation with patients about their preferences, less time to negotiate with them about what their contribution might be to the care process and greater expectation that patients should simply co-operate or comply with prescribed treatments. In the following case study one nurse finds a way to incorporate greater person-centred consultation with patients in a busy ward.

Case study: Introducing a way to collaborate with patients

Serena is a second-year nursing student on placement in a surgical ward. In reflecting on her experience, she describes how a great deal of pre- and post-operative nursing care has involved carefully following standardised procedures in a predominantly medical model of care. She feels it has encouraged a task-orientated approach to ensure that vital observations of patients and procedures are carried out, and that this can distract nurses from providing patient-centred care.

Serena noted that after patients had been given lunch the nurses usually sat down to update individualised care plans for those for whom they were responsible. Serena says, 'I like to go round the beds to ask each person if there is anything they would like me to include in their records about how they are progressing and about any concerns or preferences they might have; and by listening and looking at each person I get a mental picture of how they are feeling and what care they might need.'

In the ward where Serena was working, it was not customary practice for nurses to check with each patient before writing up the notes. Many nurses were happy to take the weight off their feet after a busy morning, and recording their observations and activities provided an opportunity for this (once patients' most pressing needs had been addressed). Serena used her initiative by inviting patients' contributions in updating their care plans as it gave her an opportunity to interact with them, which she liked; it enabled her to observe or assess them more closely, and she felt it was important they were involved in discussing the care they had received and plans for continuing care. In doing this, Serena respected patients' autonomy, facilitated freedom of choice and empowered them to influence their care. This case study also illustrates that ethical sensitivity (see Chapter 9) and collaborative decision-making are closely interrelated.

Activity 2.5   *Leadership and management*

Leadership and management styles determine the policies, customs and practices of nurses in clinical areas. This activity invites you to think about the implications of the case study regarding the management of change in adopting collaborative practices to enhance patient-centred care.

Please take a moment to reflect on your own clinical experience and see whether you can relate to any of the issues referred to by Serena.

- If you were a patient, would you like or dislike a nurse coming to ask you what you think about your care following your lunch? Why?
- If you were a nursing colleague of Serena, do you think you would praise or criticise her actions? Why?
- What might be obstacles to collaborative decision-making and patient-centred care?

Some possible answers to the last question are included at the end of the chapter.

Introducing and sustaining practice changes to overcome obstacles to greater collaborative decision-making and patient-centred care need effective leadership and management. Serena felt well-supported by her mentor, who admired her energy and commitment to patients and demonstrated this by emulating the way Serena consulted patients in updating their records. The ward manager also commented on the good quality of Serena's nursing notes during team meetings. This encouraged other nurses to follow suit, which they found rewarding as most of the patients appreciated feeling more involved in their own care. In terms of change theory, Serena was an adventurous innovator who took a risk in trying out a new way of updating notes that involved collaborating with patients. The mentor and ward sister were 'early adopters' who exercised leadership in supporting Serena's actions and encouraging others to try it out for themselves. Nurses adopted the change fairly quickly ('early majority'), after a longer period of deliberation ('late majority') or eventually, when the change seemed inevitable ('laggards') (Rogers, 1962). Barriers to change, such as lack of incentive (NICE, 2007a), were reduced through the mentor's and ward manager's flexible and responsive leadership, and by the nurses gaining a sense of satisfaction from adapting and developing their clinical practice. Ensuring that collaborative, shared decision-making between health professionals and patients is implemented is considered vital to improve patients' experience of care (NICE, 2012, 2013). Serena's case study indicates that she applied the '6Cs' of compassion, care, communication, competence, courage and commitment (DH, 2012a) in demonstrating how to improve patients' experience of care.

Even in areas such as mental healthcare – where, traditionally, more attention has been focused on what patients are thinking and feeling and on enabling patients to develop ways of dealing with various stressors – effective collaborative clinical decision-making can be difficult to achieve. The case study below demonstrates this, while reinforcing the benefit of having a supportive mentor.

Case study: Preventing a psychotic relapse

Franco is a third-year student on placement with a community mental health team. One of his responsibilities has been to help run a clinic giving long-acting anti-psychotic 'depot' injections to stabilise patients diagnosed with schizophrenia so that they can live in the community. Martin, a patient delegated to Franco by his mentor, has a history of psychotic behaviour. If he does not take his medication, he has been known to believe he is 'John the Baptist' and walk naked through town to 'cleanse the souls of sinners' or try to 'fly to heaven' and fall from an upstairs window, breaking his arm. Despite agreeing to come to the clinic, Martin repeatedly fails to attend. Franco alerts his mentor, and they do a home visit to administer the injection, which involves getting past Martin's sometimes hostile and paranoid mother (who thinks they are poisoning her son). Martin reassures her, saying, 'It's alright Mum. I'll have the injection.' He apologises for not making the clinic, saying he didn't feel like going. Franco offers to go with him to the clinic next time, but Martin says he'd rather have the injection at home. They chat about philosophy for a while as both share an interest in it. Franco leaves feeling frustrated, as he thinks Martin would benefit from getting out more and talking to other people, and he is disappointed he has failed to help him do this.

Franco's mentor asks him to visualise what might have happened if he had not alerted him that Martin had missed his appointment and they had not followed up by seeing him at home. Franco accepts he played his part in ensuring Martin's psychotic symptoms remain controlled. The mentor then praises Franco for his commitment to helping Martin, his ability to talk to him about things the mentor does not know much about and his resourcefulness in trying to negotiate a new way of getting Martin out of the house to attend the clinic. They also reflect on how seeing the home situation supports Gregory Bateson's theory about dysfunctional 'double-bind' relationships sometimes found between parents and patients prone to schizophrenia (Gibney, 2006). The mentor points out that while the mother may not seem 'normal', she has never required compulsory treatment and that her suspicions are those of an anxious mother being protective of her son. Acknowledging this and reassuring her that the injection is good for Martin can help to gain her co-operation.

Whichever field of nursing you are studying and practising in, you, like Franco, are likely to face challenges in collaborating with patients and families; having a supportive mentor will be helpful in this respect. Activity 2.6 asks you to reflect on related issues you have come across.

Activity 2.6   *Reflection*

Take a moment to think about any difficulties that you have experienced in collaborating with patients and their families. Describe the circumstances as well as you can and then examine the reasons for it. See if you can think of a new way to consult and negotiate with those concerned to gain their co-operation in achieving previously agreed aims or new revised aims.

As this is for you to review your own experience, there is no answer included, but please discuss your responses with your mentor.

The important contribution that patients and relatives make to person-centred, collaborative care is recognised in the Expert Patients Programme (DH, 2006; ORCIC and DBIS, 2013). This is where patients, particularly those with long-term conditions, are seen as 'experts' in understanding and managing their own care needs. It is acknowledged that health professionals lack understanding of what it is like to live with long-term illness or disability. The programme enables expert patients to inform, advise, support and collaborate with other patients in finding ways to cope with similar problems. In a sense, all patients are experts on their personal experience of ill health and the care that they receive so there should be *no decision about me, without me* (DH, 2012b). This is why collaborative clinical decision-making between nurses and patients is vital in order to ensure that care is truly patient-centred.

Collaborating with health professionals and other agencies

As with collaborative decision-making with patients, the need for nurses to recognise the important contribution of other health professionals in person/patient-centred care is also emphasised by the NMC in the 'Practise effectively' section of *The Code*:

8 Work co-operatively

To achieve this you must:

8.1 respect the skills, expertise and contributions of your colleagues, referring matters to them where appropriate

8.2 maintain effective communication with colleagues

8.3 keep colleagues informed when you are sharing the care of individuals with other healthcare professionals and staff

8.4 work with colleagues to evaluate the quality of your work and that of the team

8.5 work with colleagues to preserve the safety of those receiving care

8.6 share information to identify and reduce risk, and

8.7 be supportive of colleagues who are encountering health or performance problems. However, this support must never compromise or be at the expense of patient or public safety
(NMC, 2015, p8)

Collaborative clinical decision-making complements health policy to integrate patient-centred health and social care, hospital services and community services more effectively, to raise efficiency and quality and to reduce errors associated with fragmented care (DH, 2013a). It is, therefore, important to understand the roles of other health professionals and refer patients to them who need their expertise. The use of integrated care pathways (ICPs) as structured, evidence-based, multidisciplinary care plans to guide high quality care for specific clinical conditions (Campbell et al., 1998) is an example of how to acknowledge, harness and co-ordinate the contributions of different health professionals. Chapter 5 discusses ICPs in more detail. Without collaborative clinical decision-making: (i) care is not responsive to patients' or the wider public's expressed needs; (ii) different health professionals, social care and other agencies work in isolation from one another (even when attending to the same patient); (iii) there is a lack of communication, integration and co-ordination of services that they provide; (iv) necessary referrals are not made; and (v) sadly, sometimes tragically, poor quality care is likely to result from this. The case study below explores these issues.

> ## Case study: Tragic outcome of non-collaboration
>
> *In 2007 the bodies of a 38-year-old woman and her 18-year-old daughter were found in the woman's car after she is believed to have set it alight. The woman had borderline learning difficulties, and her daughter had severe learning difficulties, with an estimated mental age of just 4. They were stigmatised because of the daughter's obvious disability, and they suffered years of sustained hate, abuse, persecution and terror day and night from gangs of local youths. In the year before they died, the mother complained to the police thirteen times, but no action was taken against the offenders or to help the mother when she expressed suicidal intentions if the abuse did not stop.*
>
> *In the aftermath of the tragedy it was concluded that serious failures had occurred in: not prioritising the complaint; treating each complaint separately and not recognising the persistent pattern of abuse; not sharing information between agencies (police, social services, council housing officers); not referring the mother to get medical or nursing help to relieve the burden of caring for her daughter; and not referring her for a mental health assessment when she said she was going to kill herself because she could not cope any more.*

In this case study there was no collaborative decision-making. If there had been, the tragedy could have been prevented. When the mother repeatedly consulted the police, they did not make an adequate risk assessment, no effective strategy was negotiated to address her concerns and there was no co-operation with health and social care agencies, who were not alerted. It is one of many tragedies in recent years where the most vulnerable people in society have been let down by a lack of responsive, collaborative and integrated care (focused on the person's needs and preferences) by health and social care agencies in hospital or in the community. It is a reminder for nurses, other health and social care professionals and for community agencies that further tragedies will happen if there is no effective safety net of collaborative decision-making. Sometimes, as nurses, we could do more to let other agencies know what different skills and services we can offer patients. For example, other professions have said that they value the contribution of the community learning disability nursing service (Powell and Murray, 2004). If a referral had been made to support the family in the case study, the outcome might have been different. This reinforces calls for greater provision of and accessibility to skilled community learning disability nurses in a wide range of settings, including police referrals (RCN, 2014b).

It is probable that each of the health and social care and community agencies implicated in recent tragedies will have had a mission statement committed to providing a high quality service to all members of the public regardless of age, gender, ethnicity, culture or religion. Very often statistics are used to suggest that these organisations are being effective in the vast number of cases they deal with. The main strength of collaborative clinical decision-making in nursing is that it reminds us we are dealing with human beings who have a complex range of continually changing needs that may only be partially represented or addressed by mission statements or the science of decision analysis. In this sense, nursing theory – by focusing on good interpersonal relationships, addressing bio-psycho-social-spiritual needs and offering compassionate human caring – remains highly relevant in clinical decision-making.

Quality care through collaboration

If we do not collaborate adequately with service users, we cannot: (i) make accurate assessments of their health problems; (ii) ensure they are informed and consent to proposed care; (iii) know what their needs and preferences are; or (iv) know what their experience of the healthcare provided is. If we do not collaborate adequately with the healthcare team or other agencies, we cannot contribute to the delivery of effective, integrated, high quality, inter-professional care. Collaborative decision-making by service users and healthcare team members is, therefore, vital for high quality care.

Integrating collaboration with patients, families and other health professionals

In clinical practice nurses have to collaborate simultaneously with patients, their families, other health professionals and various agencies all the time because complex health problems need a co-ordinated approach. This is illustrated in the following case study.

> ### Case study: Collaborating with child, parents and healthcare team
>
> *Sanjeev is a seven-year-old boy who has been admitted to a children's ward in great pain and distress, having broken his arm falling from a bouncy castle at his friend's birthday party. Alison, a third-year student, welcomes him and his parents to the ward and asks a couple of other children to come and say hello. Alison asks Sanjeev to tell her what happened and where it hurts, without touching his arm in order not to exacerbate his pain. She can see that the left forearm is crooked and that there are no bones protruding through the skin, which is consistent with a 'greenstick' fracture. Alison tells Sanjeev he is very brave and clever to use his right arm to support and protect the left one, and that she will ask the doctor to see him so they can mend his arm and stop it hurting.*
>
> *X-rays confirm fractures to the radius and ulna bones in the left arm. Alison applies an anaesthetic skin patch to Sanjeev's right arm so that he won't feel the needle when given an anaesthetic before surgery. The parents try to comfort Sanjeev, but he screams and fights against the injection, so the anaesthetist gives gas via a face mask; Sanjeev inhales and loses consciousness, so they can proceed with surgery. Alison can see the parents are upset and talks to them. They express remorse for letting*
>
> *(Continued)*

continued . . .

him go to the party, not realising it had an unsupervised bouncy castle that caused their son such a serious injury. They are also sorry they could not calm Sanjeev down during the anaesthesia when he was so frightened.

Alison informs them that these injuries are common, young bones are usually quick to heal, Sanjeev will be given pain relief after surgery and he can go home in a day or two once they are sure there are no after-effects from the anaesthetic or complications with the arm or its protective cast. She shows them the family area where they can sit down and have a cup of tea while they are waiting. She mentions how they felt during the anaesthesia to her mentor, who asks her to tell the anaesthetist when surgery is over, which, nervously, she does. The anaesthetist then goes to see the parents to explain that although they try to be as gentle as possible, it is not unusual for a frightened child in a lot of pain to be resistant. But the operation went well, Sanjeev is now alert, his pain is controlled and they can go and see him.

In this case study, Alison demonstrated effective collaborative clinical decision-making with patients, families and other health professionals by consulting with:

- Sanjeev in identifying the nature and cause of his injury;
- the parents in acknowledging and reporting their concerns, and in keeping them informed so they would know how to support their son;
- the inter-professional healthcare team (nurse mentor, orthopaedic doctor, radiographer and anaesthetist) in caring for Sanjeev and diagnosing and treating his broken arm.

In doing so, Alison showed how to link theory and practice in relating caring, holistic and inter-personal values, knowledge and skills to collaborative clinical decision-making.

Sometimes you might be worried that your own role is less clear or possibly threatened by the roles and expertise of other professionals. One way of assessing the relevance of nurses' expertise within inter-professional care is to summarise the key elements of nursing and then cross-reference these with the case study examples of collaborative clinical decision-making. As mentioned in Chapter 1, nurses identified ten conceptions of nursing (plus ten perceptions of decision-making) in a research study (Standing, 2005, 2007, 2010a). They are called conceptions rather than concepts as they represent nurses' own growing understanding of their professional identity acquired through experience, as opposed to purely academic, theoretical knowledge.

Table 2.1 sets out the conceptions of nursing that Alison was applying in her care of Sanjeev and how they relate to collaborative decision-making.

Table 2.1 suggests that key characteristics (conceptions of nursing) identified by nurses (in putting into words the nature of their own professional identity) complement the integrated collaborative decision-making with patient/family and health professionals in the case study. Activity 2.7 invites you to apply the same process to your experience of healthcare teamwork.

Conceptions of nursing	Collaborative clinical decision-making
Caring	Comforting Sanjeev by telling him he is brave and clever.
Listening and being there	Enabling Sanjeev to explain how he was injured. Enabling parents to talk about their feelings.
Practical procedures	Undertaking pre-operative procedures, e.g. anaesthetic gel skin patch.
Knowledge and understanding	Pain control, pre/post-operative care, care of broken arm, developmental psychology; excluding non-accidental injury.
Communicating	Talking softly to Sanjeev, introducing him to other children; orientating parents to ward, explaining care plan and prognosis.
Patience	Remaining calm when Sanjeev is screaming and fighting off attempts to give him an intravenous anaesthetic.
Teamwork	Making referral to orthopaedic surgeon, arranging X-ray, reporting parents' concerns to mentor and to the anaesthetist.
Paperwork and electronic record	Ensuring parents have signed consent form before surgery.
Empathising and non-judgemental	Appreciating Sanjeev's distress at his painful injury when he was supposed to be having fun at a party; understanding the parents' guilt feelings, anger and concerns.
Professional	Being courteous to parents/colleagues; making competent assessment of injury; being conscientious and diligent in caring for family.

Table 2.1: Integrating collaborative clinical decision-making with conceptions of nursing

Activity 2.7   *Teamwork*

Identify an example from your own area of practice as a nurse collaborating with patients and relatives plus other health professionals. Use the same format as Table 2.1 to draw up your own table and try to match and integrate your examples of collaborative decision-making with the conceptions of nursing. Reflect on whether it is useful to relate ideas about what nursing is to collaborative decisions nurses make with other healthcare professionals.

As this is for your own personal reflection there is no outline answer included, but it might be interesting for you to ask colleagues in practice/other nursing students to work through the same activity and then compare notes.

Hopefully, you will have found that Activity 2.7 has helped to reinforce the importance of good teamwork for effective, collaborative decision-making with patients, families and other health professionals. You may also have found that cross-referencing conceptions of nursing helps you to illustrate and validate your own developing professional identity while working together with others. The caring, listening and being there, communicating, teamwork and empathising/non-judgemental conceptions marry closely to the perception of collaborative decision-making identified by nurses in research (Standing, 2005, 2007, 2010a). This is supported by health policy promoting the 6Cs of compassionate care (DH, 2012a), by higher levels of patient satisfaction where they collaborate in shared decision-making (NICE, 2012, 2013), by the RCN's emphasis upon nurses' partnership working (RCN, 2014a) and by the NMC's requirement for nurses to work co-operatively in prioritising people's needs (NMC, 2015). The ten conceptions of nursing will also be cross-referenced when reflecting on the remaining nine perceptions of clinical decision-making skills in Chapters 3–11.

Chapter summary

Of all the different perceptions of clinical decision-making identified by nurses, collaborative decision-making received the most support (Standing, 2005, 2007, 2010a). It therefore seemed the logical place to begin our exploration of nurses' clinical decision-making in this book. This chapter argued that collaborative clinical decision-making involves consultation, negotiation and co-operation with patients, relatives, inter-professional colleagues and other agencies. There may also be collaboration between patients; for example, 'expert' patients may share experience to help others' self-care. The main strengths of collaborative clinical decision-making are in promoting preventative and responsive, relevant, high quality and integrated patient/person-centred care through a good nurse–patient relationship and effective teamwork. Weaknesses include collusion, a negative type of collaboration; for example, by not helping vulnerable people we are colluding with those who abuse them. We discussed how to apply collaborative clinical decision-making, first with patients and their families and then with other health professionals; finally, we looked at how to combine them in providing high quality, integrated inter-professional healthcare. In doing so, the nature of our own professional identity as nurses was outlined, and this was shown to be well-suited and equipped for collaborative clinical decision-making and applying the '6Cs' of compassionate care (DH, 2012a).

Activities: brief outline answers

Activity 2.1: Decision-making (page 22)

You may have identified the following aspects of collaborative decision-making.

- Joint decision between two or more people.
- Identification of a shared aim.

- Working together to achieve the aim.
- Consultation, negotiation and co-operation.

Activity 2.2: Reflection (page 23)

You may have reflected on the following aspects of collusion.

- Secretive alliance promoting alternative agenda.
- Inconsistency between stated beliefs and actions.
- Actions undermining prevailing social or moral values.
- Lack of confidence to challenge inappropriate behaviour.

Activity 2.4: Communication (page 27)

You may have identified the following aspects of consulting with patients.

- Focusing attention on patients rather than on your own need for a chat.
- Eliciting views and preferences regarding patients' health needs.
- Engaging patients in collaborative clinical decision-making.
- Informing patient-centred care that is relevant to their needs.
- Explaining treatment options, enabling patients' informed consent.
- Answering patients' questions and giving health promotion advice.

Activity 2.5: Leadership and management (page 29)

You may have referred to the following obstacles to collaborative decision-making.

- Pressurised clinical environment encourages task-orientated care.
- Standardised procedures may be used to support a medical model of care.
- Fatigue may result in nurses lacking energy to talk with patients.
- Talking to patients might be seen as shirking other responsibilities.
- Nurses may not feel confident in communicating with patients.
- Collaborative decision-making is not customary practice in that area.

Further reading

Ellis, P and Bach, S (2015) *Leadership, management and team working in nursing* (2nd edn). London: Sage/Learning Matters.

Practical guide in how to get team members to work together in meeting agreed care needs of their patients.

McCormack, B and McCance, T (eds) (2016) *Person-centred practice in nursing and healthcare: theory and practice* (2nd edn). Oxford: Wiley/Blackwell.

Shows how person-centred practice involves patients participating in decisions in various healthcare settings.

Northway, R and Jenkins, R (2017) *Safeguarding adults in nursing practice* (2nd edn). London: Sage/Learning Matters.

Chapter 8 emphasises the importance of inter-professional collaboration in working with vulnerable adults.

Thomas, J, Pollard, K and Sellman, D (eds) (2014) *Interprofessional working in health and social care: professional perspectives* (2nd edn). Houndmills: Palgrave/Macmillan.

Describes inter-professional collaboration between different agencies (including police) and service users.

Useful websites

www.england.nhs.uk/nursingvision

NHS website prioritising person-centred collaborative practice within a culture of compassionate care with useful resources/downloads regarding the '6Cs' and how they can be applied in different pathways.

www.www.expertpatients.co.uk

Enables patients to access resources provided by expert patients to help them with problem solving and decision-making in managing their own long-term care needs (also useful for health professionals).

www.selfmanagementuk.org/programmes

Similar to above 'expert patients' website promoting self-management through collaboration and information sharing between more and less experienced service users and with other agencies in the community.

Chapter 3
Using observation to inform decisions

NMC Standards for Pre-registration Nursing Education

This chapter will address the following competencies:

Domain 2: Communication and interpersonal skills

4. All nurses must recognise when people are anxious or in distress and respond effectively, using therapeutic principles, to promote their wellbeing, manage personal safety and resolve conflict. They must use effective communication strategies and negotiation techniques to achieve best outcomes, respecting the dignity and human rights of all concerned. They must know when to consult a third party and how to make referrals for advocacy, mediation or arbitration.

Domain 3: Nursing practice and decision-making

7. All nurses must be able to recognise and interpret signs of normal and deteriorating mental and physical health and respond promptly to maintain or improve the health and comfort of the service user, acting to keep them and others safe.

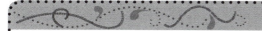

NMC Essential Skills Clusters

This chapter will address the following ESCs:

Cluster: Care, compassion and communication

6. People can trust the newly registered graduate nurse to engage therapeutically and actively listen to their needs and concerns, responding using skills that are helpful, providing information that is clear, accurate, meaningful and free from jargon.

Cluster: Organisational aspects of care

9. People can trust the newly registered graduate nurse to treat them as partners and work with them to make a holistic and systematic assessment of their needs; to develop a personalised plan that is based on mutual understanding and respect for their individual situation promoting health and wellbeing, minimising risk of harm and promoting their safety at all times.

10. People can trust the newly registered graduate nurse to deliver nursing interventions and evaluate their effectiveness against the agreed assessment and care plan.

(Continued)

continued . . .

11. People can trust the newly registered graduate nurse to safeguard children and adults from vulnerable situations and support and protect them from harm.

17. People can trust the newly registered graduate nurse to work safely under pressure and maintain the safety of service users at all times.

Chapter aims

By the end of this chapter, you should be able to:

- explain how observations inform clinical decision-making;
- give examples of decisions informed by patient observation;
- apply observation to detect physical and psychological signs;
- relate observation to patient assessment and evaluating care;
- use observation in recognising and responding to health risks;
- appreciate the importance of observation in decision-making.

Introduction

Without observation, patient-centred clinical judgement and decision-making in evidence-based nursing care is not possible. For example, collaborative decision-making (Chapter 2) relies upon good observation: nurses need to be attentive to what patients tell them and healthcare colleagues need to share observations of patients' health status. We cannot assess what patients' problems are without observing them and we cannot tell whether there is any change in their condition without observing them. It is therefore vital for nurses to develop effective observational skills to inform decisions regarding patient assessment, care planning and evaluation of care. The significance of observations also needs to be understood in order to decide what action needs to be taken to resolve the issues identified. In the research study that informs this book (Standing, 2005, 2007, 2010a), one nursing student's personal account closely relates observation to the role of the nurse in clinical decision-making, as shown below.

Case study: Destined to be a nurse

When asked to reflect on reasons why she had chosen to study nursing, Serena described an early childhood memory where she had recognised that another child needed medical attention.

'When I was seven I was playing outside my home and I saw a neighbour's child fall down as he was running across the road. He had sliced open the skin underneath his chin, which had hit the kerb as

continued . . .

> he fell, and it was bleeding. The boy looked unsteady when he got up and he was crying. There were grown-ups who saw what happened and lots of other children around but everyone seemed to be in a panic. I just grabbed the kid, held him under the chin and walked with him to see his mother. So people said, "She's a nurse" and it's just stuck from that moment.'

Serena's childhood memory nicely illustrates the importance of **observation in clinical decision-making**, and how an ability to link the two is associated with being a nurse by members of the public. Observation is important because without it you cannot see if anything is wrong with a person. However, it is limited unless followed by appropriate judgement, decision-making and action to address the problem by relieving pain or suffering, and promoting healing and recovery. For example, the 'grown-ups' saw what had happened to the boy but did not take any action. Perhaps they did not think the injury was as serious as Serena thought, and if she had not intervened, the boy might have made his own way home to be cared for by his mother. Knowing whether to act on observations in healthcare is therefore very much a 'judgement call'.

Serena showed how observation can be effectively used to inform decision-making by:

- being alert to changing situations and any associated health risks;
- recognising that the boy was distressed and nobody was helping him;
- remaining calm in responding and attending to the boy after the accident;
- assessing the boy's physical injury and his emotional reaction;
- applying first aid to minimise blood loss by supporting his chin;
- transferring the boy to his mother for further treatment and comfort;
- reporting observations and reasons for decisions and actions;
- exercising leadership, inspiring others to have confidence in her.

This chapter explores nurses' use of observation to inform decisions, starting by clarifying what this entails and its relevance to evidence-based nursing. Observation of patients' physical and mental health is described, and examples of assessment and evaluating care are given. The use of observation is explored in relation to risk assessment and management, including 'track and trigger' early warning systems where a rapid response may be needed. The importance of accurately recording observations is then emphasised. Finally, the strengths and weaknesses of using observation to inform decisions are summarised.

What does using observation to inform decisions mean?

Observation is usually associated with using our eyes in noticing what is happening around us, just as Serena did when she saw the boy fall. We also use other senses to get information about situations we find ourselves in; for example, if Serena had not seen the boy fall, she would still have known something was wrong because she could hear him crying. Blind or partially sighted people rely more on hearing, feeling their way around using a white stick or being accompanied by a guide dog or a sighted companion. Conversely, the deaf or partially deaf compensate by relying more on sight in 'lip reading' and using sign language. Those of us fortunate to have good eyesight and hearing can learn from those with sensory impairment by making fuller use of the senses we possess. For example, we can emulate deaf people by paying closer attention to 'body language' when interacting with others, just as Serena did when recognising the boy was distressed and others 'seemed to be in a panic'. We also use the senses of smell and taste every day – when we are judging whether our food or drink is safe to consume, for example. If a patient's breath smells strongly of acetone (i.e. like nail polish), this is an indication they may be in danger of going into a diabetic coma due to lack of insulin. Detecting and reporting this would ensure that urgent medical care could be given as necessary. Observation is not restricted to what we can see; it involves the use of all the senses in processing stimuli.

At any one time our senses are being continually bombarded by a wide range of stimuli, even if we are sitting quietly trying to read. Many of these sensory stimuli go unnoticed as they are filtered out of consciousness because they are deemed irrelevant to the task at hand. This can be helpful and unhelpful in relation to decision-making. For example, your decision to try to learn something useful by reading this chapter is helped if you are able to ignore distractions such as a neighbour playing heavy metal music at full volume. On the other hand, being unaware of how to control distractions is unhelpful, as you are less likely to be successful at completing the tasks you set yourself. Observation skills are useful for knowing how to focus attention on important things and for recognising, and avoiding where possible, unhelpful stimuli that are an unnecessary distraction. Sometimes it is important to be distracted from what you are doing – it is clearly unwise to carry on reading if you smell burning, see smoke and hear the fire alarm. What is considered to be a priority can, therefore, suddenly change. As nurses caring for patients, we need to be even more vigilant in developing and applying the observation skills needed to accurately inform decisions that promote health and minimise risks.

Relevance of observation in evidence-based nursing

For the purposes of this chapter, observation means:

> *using all the senses (sight, hearing, touch, smell, taste) to assess patients' bio-psycho-social-spiritual health and wellbeing, check if they need assistance, monitor their vital signs, review results of investigations, record response to treatment and report concerns.*

As we saw in Chapter 1, observation skills have historically been associated with nursing. For example, Florence Nightingale demonstrated and advocated their use in showing that increased survival rates following surgery were associated with improvements in hygiene and sanitation. Similarly, the nursing process relies upon nurses' accurate observations to assess patients' problems and evaluate the effects of nursing interventions. More recently, the promotion of evidence-based practice has posed questions about the accuracy of nursing perceptions and observations. The intention behind this policy is to promote high quality care that is based upon sound research evidence, as opposed to local custom and practice that may fail to keep up with new developments. While it makes sense to be aware of potential errors, it results in 'throwing the baby out with the bathwater' if our observations of patients are no longer considered relevant. It is good to update knowledge ('throw bathwater') but not good to de-skill nurses or undermine professional identity ('throw baby') developed by *observing* and interacting with patients. This chapter argues that observation is a vital part of well-informed, patient-centred, evidence-based nursing.

The Code specifying nurses' professional standards of conduct states, *Always practise in line with the best available evidence* (NMC, 2015, p7). The idea that some forms of evidence might be considered better than others (in terms of being more rigorously researched or tested) has led to the development of hierarchies of evidence such as the one shown in Table 3.1. This assumes that level 1 is the strongest and level 7 the weakest type of evidence in the range.

A quick look at Table 3.1 indicates that nursing observations do not feature as a specific form of evidence in the hierarchy although, arguably, level 7 may be informed by expert nurses' observations. Observation is vital in carrying out research referred to in levels 1–6; otherwise there would be no results to report, and no research-based NICE (National Institute of Health and Care Excellence) clinical guidelines published. However, research observations differ from nursing observations: the main focus is to generate knowledge rather than deliver care; they are constrained by the specific research questions being asked; and it is often recommended that the results are applied to other areas that were not observed or included in the research study. The hierarchy prompts nurses to value research observations from elsewhere as more reliable types of evidence than their own observations of patient care.

Level	Evidence source
1	Systematic review of experimental research studies that used randomised controlled trials (RCTs)
2	At least one randomised controlled trial
3	'Quasi' experimental research study using a non-randomised controlled trial
4	Non-experimental research such as case control and cohort studies or randomised surveys
5	Systematic review of descriptive or qualitative research (e.g. non-randomised surveys, case studies)
6	At least one descriptive or qualitative research study
7	Expert opinion and reports from authoritative committees

Table 3.1: A hierarchy of evidence – relative value of external sources of evidence (1 = highest, 7 = lowest)
Source: Adapted from Melnyk and Fineout-Overholt (2014)

This can place nurses in a bit of a quandary as we are required to be observant, attentive and responsive in giving relevant 'person-centred care' (NMC, 2010, 2015) while, wherever possible, applying rigorous research evidence that has not directly involved the patients we are caring for. Being both patient-centred and evidence-based can seem like trying to 'fit a square peg into a round hole' if nursing observations are not considered a valid form of evidence, or if in applying research findings, patients' individual needs and preferences are not addressed. Activity 3.1 asks you to think about how observation skills contributed to Serena's decision-making in the case study and whether her actions are supported by more authoritative sources of evidence.

Activity 3.1   *Decision-making*

Hint: Remember that decision-making involves choosing a course of action from the available options, an ability to explain the reasoning behind it and being accountable for the outcome.

Look back at the description of the case study where Serena helped the boy who had hurt himself, and try to answer the following questions.

1. How did Serena know that anything was wrong?
2. What were the different options available to Serena?
3. Why do you think she chose to intervene as described?
4. How might Serena's actions have affected the boy's recovery?
5. What theory or research might support Serena's decision-making?

There are some possible answers at the end of the chapter.

Now that you have completed Activity 3.1, we should be 'on the same page' in that you can see that observations we make about people in our care are vital sources of evidence. If we do not act on these observations, patients can suffer harm, which could potentially be fatal. It may seem a bit odd that the carer in the case study is so young, and you might, understandably, feel reluctant to compare your skills and experience with those of a seven-year-old. However, it makes the point that someone with no professional education in healthcare is able to recognise the need to respond to an emergency, and to do so in an appropriate manner (even if she was unable to explain the first aid principles (SJA et al., 2016) she applied). This reinforces the importance of our own observations as nurses in caring for people and how they contribute to our professional knowledge and skills, in addition to formal education, theory and research.

As students you might also expect (as Serena did) that more experienced people – for example, your clinical mentor – will know what to do and guide you in facing challenging situations.

Decision-making requires more than knowing what to do in a given situation – you also need to know why you are taking a particular action, and be able to explain and justify it. This is where we need to link theory and practice by relating our nursing observations and experience to theoretical principles and more scientific forms of evidence. Your mentors and role models will demonstrate how to do this, and as you progress through your programme you will find it easier to integrate theory and practice in this respect. In doing so you will discover a way to resolve the quandary of being attentive and responsive in giving localised, patient-centred care and, at the same time, ensure that up-to-date relevant national and international research evidence is applied to practice.

In summary, we can 'change the bathwater without losing the baby' and find a way of making 'square pegs' and 'round holes' more compatible, by acknowledging the following points:

- Nursing observations are valid forms of evidence to inform decision-making because they are patient-centred and enable us to quickly assess and respond to health risks.
- Research evidence is rigorously developed and tested accumulated knowledge that goes beyond that found via personal or local experience, to inform healthcare decisions.
- Nursing observations can be enhanced by applying research evidence in relation to the different assessment/decision-making tools or clinical treatment guidelines we can use.
- Research evidence will remain 'on the library shelf' unless nursing observations are used to identify its relevance to inform and support our decision-making in patient-centred care.

There is a growing understanding that various forms of evidence have to be acknowledged because different types of problems or circumstances call for different types of knowledge and skills to be applied (Rycroft-Malone et al., 2004; Rolfe et al., 2008). This challenges the concept of a hierarchy because each type of evidence has its own strengths and applications; for example, non-experimental methods such as qualitative research offer more in-depth understanding of people's experience than randomised controlled trials. In addition to the evidence shown in Table 3.1, Ellis (2016) identifies practice knowledge, experience and patient preference as important influences in evidence-based nursing decisions, all incorporating nurses observing, listening to and interacting with patients. Hence, observation skills are vital in care which is both patient-centred and evidence-based. In relating the principles of evidence-based practice to systematic **problem solving** in patient-centred nursing care, Moule (2015) describes five key stages. These are summarised below with a nursing example to show how they might be applied.

1. Identify a nursing problem and make it into a specific question (e.g. patient prescribed large tablets cannot swallow them – is there an alternative way to give the medicine?).
2. Search literature/other sources to find the answer to your question (talk to mentor, who advises you to check whether the British National Formulary (BNF) has information on this).
3. Critically evaluate rigour and relevance of the evidence you find (find up-to-date edition of BNF which indicates the medicine can also be given in syrup form).
4. Select and apply best evidence to address patient need/preference (tell doctor of problem and possible solution; doctor agrees to prescribe syrup so patient can take medicine).
5. Evaluate patient outcome after the evidence-based intervention (patient is able to swallow the syrup and is happy that an alternative to the tablets has been found).

Systematic problem solving and decision-making in nursing is discussed in more detail in Chapter 4. In the meantime, to help you self-assess how much sense you make of what has been discussed so far, Activity 3.2 asks you to think about how nursing observations might contribute to evidence-based practice using the five stages referred to by Moule.

Activity 3.2   *Evidence-based practice and research*

Hint: Assess what each stage does plus their collective contribution to patient-centred care.

Look at Moule's five stages of evidence-based practice and answer these questions.

1. Which stages are more strongly associated with nursing observations and why?
2. What do you need to do to access evidence that helps tackle nursing problems?
3. How is research or other evidence nurses find related to patient-centred care?

There are some possible answers at the end of the chapter.

For the purposes of this book, evidence-based practice means:

> *never being satisfied you 'know it all' and using critical thinking skills to continually search, access, critique and apply the most relevant up-to-date sources of information to guide clinical judgement/decision-making in giving the highest quality patient-centred care possible, and evaluating the results.*

In discussing the relevance of observation to evidence-based nursing, it was argued that nurses' observations are valid forms of evidence in their own right and that they enable us to identify, apply and evaluate other evidence, including research, in patient-centred care. Nursing observations are a window into the world of the patients we care for and interact with, using all of our senses.

Research evidence is a window into the wider world of accumulated current knowledge that we tap into to develop our knowledge and understanding, and to enhance the quality of care we give patients. Other types of evidence also inform our practice, including feedback from patients, peers, mentors and inter-professional colleagues, informative textbooks and relevant clinical guidelines. **Evidence** is, therefore, any kind of information that is used to support reasoning, problem solving, clinical judgement and decision-making, including nursing observations, feedback from patients and colleagues, clinical guidelines, health policy, relevant theory and research findings.

Observations used to monitor physical health

As human beings, our capacity to sustain life is dependent on our ability to address biological needs, including breathing, maintaining blood flow to all our major organs, eating and drinking, eliminating waste, protecting ourselves from injury or disease, exercising and resting. All these activities can be monitored in patients in our care through nursing observations, enabling us to decide whether any intervention is necessary to help patients maintain their vital functions. In order to make accurate observations we need to learn the correct techniques and how to use relevant equipment. To appreciate the significance of the observations, we need a good understanding of relevant anatomy and physiology, and how to distinguish normal from abnormal functioning. We then have to decide whether our observations require further action, which might include double-checking results, increasing the frequency of observations, reporting changes to the clinical manager, helping a patient with heat stroke to cool down, elevating the bottom of the bed to help return blood to the heart for a patient with low blood pressure or calling for emergency help if a patient stops breathing. It is vital our observations are not considered ritualistic, routine tasks or 'ends in themselves' but as valuable sources of information to assess patients' health and guide decision-making. This is illustrated in the case study below.

Case study: Reporting alarming change in vital signs

Lucy is a second-year student nurse on an orthopaedic ward who is asked to observe and record the vital signs of the patients she is helping to care for. Miranda, aged 25, was knocked off her motorcycle by a van whose driver did not see her, and she has a hairline fracture on the back of her skull, a fractured pelvis and a compound fracture of the tibia and fibula in her left leg. Medical assessment of Miranda indicates that her skull and pelvis should heal by themselves but that nurses need to closely observe her for signs of neurological damage (e.g. eyes/pupils not reacting to light, loss of consciousness) or internal bleeding (e.g. low blood pressure, increased respiration and heart rate). Miranda's leg fractures were realigned by screwing into her tibia/shinbone pins that protrude eight centimetres from her skin and support two metal 'external fixators' (looks like leg scaffolding). Before Miranda left the operating theatre, a sterile dressing and bandage were applied to the wound (caused by fractured bones breaking through her skin during the accident).

It is now three days since surgery, and so far Miranda has been progressing reasonably well. She is nursed in bed with her left leg elevated to reduce swelling, and she has regular painkillers. Miranda's temperature has been above average (37.7–38.4 degrees centigrade). Lucy's mentor says it may be the body working overtime to heal after trauma, but it needs careful monitoring. Other vital signs are within the normal range. The next time Lucy checks Miranda's temperature she is shocked to find it is 40.8 degrees. She wonders if it is a faulty reading, although it is the same device that she has used before (infrared digital aural thermometer) that she placed in Miranda's left ear as she usually does. Lucy tries again in the right ear, and gets the same result. She asks Miranda how she feels; she replies that she feels cold, and she appears to be shivering. Lucy gets a blanket for her and brings a different infrared digital aural thermometer to double-check whether the previous device was faulty. This time the reading is 41 degrees centigrade so Lucy records it on Miranda's observation chart together with her pulse and respiration rate, which show a slight increase, and her blood pressure, which remains stable. Lucy tells her mentor about the change in Miranda's condition. The mentor confirms Miranda's temperature is 41 degrees and alerts the medical team. They decide that there is a risk Miranda's leg is infected and that it could spread to the bloodstream (septicaemia). There is also a possibility the leg may have to be amputated if the infection does not respond to treatment. They take Miranda back to theatre to thoroughly clean her leg and change the dressing in sterile conditions, and they start her on a course of intravenous antibiotics. The antibiotics are effective and the infection subsides. Miranda's leg wound heals, the tibia and fibula mend following more orthopaedic and plastic surgery, and six months later she can walk unassisted again.

The case study shows how valuable nursing observations are in early detection and treatment of potentially serious health risks to patients. Lucy did not simply check and record temperature unthinkingly; she was constantly reviewing the significance of observations she made regarding Miranda's health status, and acting upon them if they appeared unusual, as follows.

- Checking with her mentor when the earlier temperature was over one degree above average.
- Repeating digital aural thermometer readings in the other ear to check the result.
- Checking with Miranda how she felt and giving her a blanket when she was shivering.
- Checking the accuracy of the first device by using a second digital aural thermometer.
- Realising that this was a worrying development that she needed to both record and report.
- Checking with her mentor, who confirmed the current temperature was four degrees above average.
- Prompting her mentor to inform the medical team, who treated the infection, which helped the leg to heal.

This demonstrates good practice in carrying out regular observations of patients' vital signs to recognise and respond to the continually changing health status of those with acute illnesses (NICE, 2007b). If Lucy had not reported Miranda's very high temperature straight-away, the outcome might not have been so positive, as the required medical treatment would have been delayed. It emphasises the importance of nurses being vigilant in carrying out and reporting observations. They are vital in 'track and trigger' systems such as Early Warning Score (EWS), Modified Early Warning Score (MEWS), Paediatric Early Warning Score (PEWS) and National Early Warning Score (NEWS) where increased levels of observation and intervention (e.g. medical referral) are prompted when specified thresholds are reached (e.g. very high/very low temperature, blood pressure, pulse or respiration rate). NICE recommends that all acutely ill patients in general hospital settings have the following vital signs recorded at least twelve-hourly in order to detect possible problems early on so that appropriate action can be taken.

Key vital signs	Adult normal range
Heart rate	60–100 beats per minute (bpm)
Respiratory rate	10–20 bpm
Systolic blood pressure	100–140 mmHg
Level of consciousness	Alert and responsive
Oxygen saturation	94–100% SpO_2
Temperature	36.1–37.2 degrees Celsius

Where the NEWS system is being used, each of the above areas of observation is given a score, ranging from 0 to 3 in relation to the measurements taken. If the observation is within an agreed normal range as indicated above then it would score 0 (zero). If it is higher or lower than normal, it would score from 1 to 3 according to how much it deviates from the norm as defined in local clinical guidelines (e.g. heart rate greater than 130 bpm, respiratory rate greater than 30 bpm, systolic blood pressure 70 mmHg or less and oxygen saturation 86% SpO_2

or less each score the maximum 3). The scores for each observation are added together to give a NEWS score. If the total NEWS score is only 1 there would be no need to increase the frequency of observations from the twelve-hourly minimum.

If the NEWS score increases, it should trigger an escalation activity, including increased levels of observation and intervention in order to manage increased risks to patients' health and wellbeing, and prevent further deterioration. For example, a score of 2 would trigger minimum six-hourly observations; a score of 3 would trigger minimum four-hourly observations and a medical review within an hour of the change; a score of 4–6 would trigger minimum one-hourly observations and medical review within half an hour of the change; and a score of 7 or more would trigger minimum 30-minute observations, immediate medical review, and possible activation of an Emergency Response System (ERS) (DH, 2013b). If any patient is receiving oxygen therapy they are given an extra 2 points which is added to their oxygen saturation score (RCP, 2015). As well as the aggregate scores triggering an escalation in medical and nursing care, a score of 3 in any one area (e.g. level of consciousness – unresponsive to voice or pain stimuli) requires minimum 30-minute observations and immediate medical review. Nurses are also encouraged to report any other concerns they may have about patients to the responsible medical officer promptly in case they notice something significant which may not immediately be apparent from physiological observations alone. The above 'Track and trigger' systems highlight the importance of observation skills in clinical decision-making and how observing changes in vital signs outside of normal values should result in an escalation in levels of observation and intervention in order to prevent a patient's health deteriorating wherever possible. The NEWS example relates to adults but the same principles apply to children using PEWS and COAST (Children's Observation And Severity Tool) track and trigger systems, where normal thresholds may be different from adults (e.g. heart rate is normally higher in infants and young children).

Activity 3.3   *Evidence-based practice and research*

Look at the list of nursing observations in the table below, and think of all the health risks that each one can help us identify. Then use the web/library to search for more evidence and jot down findings for future reference. Discuss with your mentor any procedures you need more practice in.

Observations	Identifying potential health risks
Temperature	
Pulse	
Respiration	
Blood pressure	
Oxygen saturation	

(Continued)

continued . . .

- Urine analysis

- Weight

- Skin appearance

- Neurological

- Pain chart

- Fluid balance

- Bowel movement

As this activity is intended to be a self-directed learning experience there is no answer provided, but you might find it useful to talk to your colleagues and compare findings.

Having looked at physical observations, we turn to those of a more elusive psychological nature.

Observations to monitor mental health

In many ways observations of mental health are less clear-cut and quantifiable than those used to monitor physical health. However, some of the observations we make of patients' physical health may be relevant when assessing mental health, as the following examples illustrate.

- Anxiety can cause the heart to beat faster than normal (tachycardia), and the person may become aware of an unusual heart rhythm (palpitations), which increases anxiety.
- Anxiety may also cause a person to breathe rapidly and shallowly (hyperventilation).
- Low body weight is sometimes due to a psychological illness called anorexia nervosa or self-neglect associated with depression, psychosis, alcohol addiction or drug addiction.
- Neurological functions (e.g. consciousness, perception, co-ordination) can be disrupted by psychotic delusions or hallucinations, intoxication or the side-effects of prescribed drugs.

As in observing physical health there are different levels of observation according to the risks associated with a patient's mental health needs. General observation (having a general idea of where patients are at all times) is for low-risk patients. Constant observation (knowing precisely where patients are as they are kept within sight of a nurse at all times) is for high-risk patients. Special observation (nurse constantly observes patient and keeps them within arm's length at all times) is for very high-risk patients who pose an imminent risk of self-harm or harming others. Mental health observations focus upon a person's mood, thoughts and behaviour.

Mood (affect)

We all experience a range of changing emotions – happy, sad, anxious, fearful or angry – in relation to the activities and life events that we are experiencing and the people we interact with.

However, getting stuck in a particular mood can result in us becoming manic, depressed, obsessive, phobic, paranoid, psychopathic, or a combination of these such as bi-polar (manic depression) illness with extreme mood swings. A person's appearance, body language, verbal expression and behaviour usually conveys their mood in a way that others can easily recognise. However, it may not always be obvious due to individual differences as some people cry when they are happy and others may smile when they are angry. We therefore also need to know about what a person is thinking when observing and assessing their mood.

Thoughts (cognition)

Who? Where? When? These are the questions asked to check how well orientated and alert a person is. Do they know who they are, where they are and when they are here (day/month/year)? If they have problems answering, the cause of their confusion needs to be established. Simply asking someone an open question about what they are thinking can sometimes help them to reveal things about themselves they would not usually volunteer. It is important that we discover if a person has a good grasp of reality or if they have any irrational beliefs such as paranoid delusions or perceptual abnormalities such as auditory hallucinations that resist any concrete evidence to the contrary. We also need to know how a person's thoughts relate to their moods in assessing risks to themselves or to others; for example, what might they think about doing when they are feeling down and depressed or frustrated and angry?

Behaviour

A person's behaviour is something we can observe more directly than their mood or thoughts. It can include how well they communicate with people, relationships with family, friends or others, work or leisure activity, sleep patterns and how well they look after their personal care. In assessing health risks we need to check if depressive feelings or paranoid thoughts were acted upon in the past, as this makes it more likely the person may harm themselves or others again. A review of research literature concluded there are five behaviours which enhance our sense of wellbeing and mental health (Aked et al., 2008; Trenoweth et al., 2011):

1. CONNECT   Maintaining network of mutually beneficial relationships with others
2. BE ACTIVE   Regular exercise (even walking) enhances physical and mental health
3. TAKE NOTICE   Attending to physical and social surroundings and how it affects you
4. KEEP LEARNING   Developing new skills gives sense of achievement/boosts confidence
5. GIVE   Helping others can be rewarding and it also takes the mind off oneself

Someone displaying all these behaviours is likely to feel good about life in general. These 'five ways to wellbeing' also increase 'mental capital' by enhancing our cognitive abilities, emotional intelligence, self-esteem and resilience in being able to find ways of coping with stressful life events (Aked et al., 2008, p13). Conversely, if a person is withdrawn and disconnected from others, inactive and lethargic (or overactive and agitated), unaware of or distracted from what's going on around them, unable to learn from past mistakes or too preoccupied with their own needs to focus upon others, they are likely to be unhappy and unfulfilled. Enabling people to develop in these areas according to their own preferences, abilities (including those with learning disabilities) and circumstances will enhance their mental health and wellbeing. Observing the above five behaviours is therefore helpful to inform mental health assessment and intervention decisions.

Activity 3.4   *Research and reflection*

This activity invites you to undertake an online self-assessment of your mood on the NHS Choices website. The purpose of the exercise is to (i) help you to appreciate what it is like for a patient undergoing mental health assessment; (ii) familiarise you with the way questions are formulated when assessing a person's mood; (iii) give you an opportunity to reflect upon and develop awareness of your own needs in this respect; (iv) develop your understanding of how questioning can enhance nursing observations and decision-making.

Go to **www.nhs.uk/conditions/stress-anxiety-depression/pages/low-mood-stress-anxiety.aspx**.

Halfway down the page on the right-hand side you will find a 'Mood Assessment' box. Click on start and answer the 18-question (multiple-choice) quiz. Please note that it is completely anonymous and you are not required to identify yourself. It is designed as a tool for members of the public to use to increase their understanding of themselves and possibly suggest ways forward in relation to the answers given.

As this is for your own personal reflection there is no outline answer included.

In the following case study, a third-year mental health nurse is on a community placement that includes monitoring the wellbeing of residents in a hostel following their discharge from a psychiatric hospital unit.

Case study: From self-neglect and social isolation to self-care and social interaction

Phillip (aged 53) has had several admissions to mental health units to be treated for depression and suicidal thoughts. He has always been very shy, and his self-confidence took a further dive when he was made redundant from a computer programming job five years ago. His wife then left him for another man. They have one grown-up son who Phillip rarely sees. Phillip now has a part-time job as a maintenance technician at an internet café near the hostel where he lives.

Jim, a third-year mental health student, visits Phillip once a week with his mentor to monitor his progress. Jim notices that Phillip's trousers look too big and discovers he has not been eating well since leaving hospital. With his mentor's agreement, Jim asks Phillip if he would like to work with him over the next eight weeks to look at ways of improving his diet.

Phillip uses his computer skills to become an expert in counting calories, nutritional properties of different foods, maximum daily levels of salt, sugar and fat to consume, and how to calculate and categorise his body

continued . . .

> *mass index to see if he is underweight, normal or overweight. He keeps in touch with Jim via email and they plan his daily menu a week in advance. Jim goes shopping with Phillip to a local general store on a couple of occasions, and Phillip finds they are quite friendly to him, and goes on his own from that point on. Jim and Phillip also experiment in the communal kitchen with tuna pasta bake, spaghetti Bolognese and chicken curry and rice. This enables Phillip to get to know the other residents better, and they begin to regard him as their 'resident boffin', answering questions about what they are eating and drinking. In exchange, they start to invite Phillip to join them if there is a good film worth watching. At the end of Jim's placement Phillip is eating better, has regained some weight and feels more self-confident, at ease with other residents.*

As mentioned earlier, physical observations often reveal aspects of a person's mental health. Jim's observation that Phillip's trousers were too big revealed that he had been neglecting his diet. This gave them both something tangible to work towards and achieve. Phillip used his computer expertise to learn new knowledge and skills, and these led to making social contact with other residents and local shopkeepers, which increased his self-confidence. This form of therapy focuses on behaviour rather than on exploring painful feelings and memories that Phillip evidently had, but that no one could really do anything about. Jim was relieved he had found something he could help Phillip with because he did not know what to say that might help him get over the painful life events he had experienced. The rationale for such activity-based therapy is that actually doing things helps to change your mood and mindset (NICE, 2009).

A key risk factor regarding Phillip's aftercare following discharge from hospital was a possibility he might get so depressed that he could act on the suicidal intentions he had previously expressed. Jim's mentor struck a balance between enabling him to develop his confidence and skills in working with Phillip 'one-to-one' and independently observing and assessing Phillip's progress to ensure any potential suicidal risk was as controlled as it could be. He also talked to Jim about plans he had made with Phillip, the effects of implementing these and the need to record everything he did, including extracts of his email exchanges, as required by the NMC:

> **10 Keep clear and accurate records relevant to your practice.**

> *This includes but is not limited to patient records. It includes all records that are relevant to your scope of practice.*
> (NMC, 2015, p9)

Activity 3.5 asks you to critique Jim's involvement in Phillip's mental healthcare.

Activity 3.5   *Critical thinking*

When discussing ways to assess or monitor a person's mental health, observations of physical signs, mood, thoughts and behaviour were identified. Using these criteria, how would you assess the progress Phillip seemed to make in the eight weeks that Jim was working with him?

Some possible answers can be found at the end of the chapter.

Table 3.2 relates the case study to observation in decision-making and conceptions of nursing.

Conceptions of nursing	Observation in clinical decision-making
Caring	Jim was concerned Phillip was not looking after himself.
Listening and being there	Jim observed that Phillip was good with computers and encouraged him to share the knowledge he had gained.
Practical procedures	Jim helped Phillip to organise menus, plan and execute shopping trips, and prepare various home-cooked meals.
Knowledge and understanding	Jim knew his limitations so he did not offer Phillip counselling, but focused instead on applying an understanding of nutrition.
Communicating	Jim questioned Phillip about his ill-fitting trousers and agreed plans to work together to address his dietary problems.
Patience	Jim committed to eight weeks of helping Phillip and understood that progress had to be at a pace Phillip was comfortable with.
Teamwork	Jim worked closely with his mentor to oversee the care given.
Paperwork and electronic record	Jim recorded the plan of care and progress in achieving goals in case notes, including an audit trail of emails with Phillip.
Empathising and non-judgemental	Jim understood Phillip had lost his job and wife, rarely saw his son and found relationships difficult, and did not blame him.
Professional	Jim realised that, despite respecting and liking Phillip, he was not his friend. He was a person it was his duty to help.

Table 3.2: Integrating observation in clinical decision-making and conceptions of nursing

The case study reveals that Jim helped Phillip develop the 'five ways to wellbeing'. Phillip became more comfortable in getting to know and interacting with the other residents (Connect); in addition to walking to his part-time job, he now regularly walks to the shops to get groceries (Be active); he has discovered that the local shopkeepers are more friendly to him than he feared (Take notice); he has learnt a lot about healthy nutrition, planning and cooking meals (Keep learning); and he is happy to answer questions from other residents when sharing his knowledge of nutrients and calories with them (Give). All of this stemmed from Jim observing that Phillip's trousers were falling down as he had lost weight, showing how nursing observations inform clinical decision-making that is both patient-centred and evidence-based.

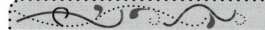

Chapter summary

This chapter argued that nursing observations are important and valid sources of evidence to inform patient-centred clinical judgement, decision-making and care delivery. It was accepted that such observations may not be as rigorously tested as some forms of research evidence. The key strength of nursing observations are that they focus on what is happening physically and psychologically to the patient, enabling their needs or preferences to be assessed, and the effects of treatment and care evaluated in relation to patient outcomes and satisfaction levels. They have potential in a preventative way to detect early warning signs and respond appropriately to avoid deterioration in patients' health. Nursing observations are also needed to identify questions about how to address patients' needs or improve the quality of care they receive in identifying, accessing, reviewing, applying relevant research results and evaluating their effects. Without nursing observations and related questions, much useful research will remain unused 'on the library shelf'. The weaknesses of nursing observations are that they are subject to individual variations in the perceptiveness of the observers and the accuracy of equipment they may use. Nursing observations are by their very nature localised, and there may be a danger of overlooking relevant research and more scientific forms of evidence that could enhance the quality of care. Hence it is necessary to apply observations systematically (as discussed in Chapter 4) to combine the benefits of patient-centred care and evidence-based nursing.

Activities: brief outline answers

Activity 3.1: Decision-making (page 44)

1. Serena saw the boy fall down, noticed that he was unsteady when he got up, that he had a significant cut underneath his chin, which was bleeding, and that he was crying.
2. Serena could have: carried on with what she was doing as she was not obliged to look after the boy; left it to the grown-ups to decide what to do; let the boy make his own way home to get help; or taken the initiative to help him herself.
3. Serena probably chose to intervene because: she recognised the boy was hurt; nobody else was helping him; he appeared to need medical attention and comforting; she knew where he lived; and she understood his mother was responsible for her son's care.
4. Serena's actions might have helped the boy to begin to recover from the injury by: supporting him under the chin in order to stem blood loss, preventing the wound from gaping, making it easier to suture (if required) and minimise potential scarring; removing him from the roadside where, in his unsteady state, he might be at risk of further injury; and reporting the accident so his mother could arrange medical assessment/treatment if necessary.
5. Serena's decision-making was consistent with the principles of first aid in: keeping calm when assessing risks; not causing any further harm; removing the boy from danger; giving early intervention; controlling blood loss; comforting the victim who might be dazed or in shock; and transferring him to an appropriate agency for continued care (SJA et al., 2016).

Activity 3.2: Evidence-based practice and research (page 46)

1. Stages 1 and 5 because they require nurses to observe patients – in order to identify problems – and to evaluate the effects of research-based interventions, respectively.
2. Identify a problem and make it into a specific question you can search for an answer to.
3. Research evidence is related to patient-centred care by: searching for evidence relevant to nursing problems; selecting evidence that helps address patients' needs/preferences; and evaluating patient outcomes regarding the effects of applying the research evidence.

Activity 3.5: Critical thinking (page 53)

Progress: physical: improved diet, put on weight, clothes fitting better.

Progress: mood: feeling more self-confident and valued by others.

Progress: thoughts: acquired new understanding and expertise regarding nutrition.

Progress: behaviour: able to plan menu, go shopping, cook meals and interact more with others.

Further reading

Blows, WT (2012) *The biological basis of clinical observations.* Abingdon: Routledge.

Contains detailed explanations about the physiological observations that inform clinical decisions.

Chambers, M (2017) *Psychiatric and mental health nursing: the craft of caring* (3rd edn). Abingdon: CRC Press.

Comprehensive, person-centred, evidence-based reference source covering a wide range of mental health issues, nursing principles and practice, including the importance of clinical observations.

Useful website

www.nice.org.uk

The National Institute for Health and Care Excellence provides freely available evidence-based clinical guidelines in caring for specific health problems, including nursing observations required in the ongoing assessment and evaluation of care within any of the adult/child/mental health/learning disability pathways.

Chapter 4
Systematic clinical decision-making

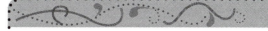

> **Chapter aims**
>
> By the end of this chapter, you should be able to:
>
> - understand, explain and apply systematic clinical decision-making;
> - describe the use of systematic decision-making in the nursing process;
> - apply the nursing process in systematically assessing the activities of living;
> - apply systematic clinical decision-making in evidence-based practice.

Introduction

So far in our exploration of clinical judgement and decision-making we have looked at nursing concepts (Chapter 1), collaborating with patients/families and healthcare teams (Chapter 2) and using observation skills to inform decisions (Chapter 3). This chapter combines and applies the different strands from earlier chapters within **systematic clinical decision-making**, a methodical, disciplined and comprehensive approach to patient-centred nursing and healthcare.

The term 'systematic' means *making use of, or carried out according to, a clearly worked-out plan or method* (Chambers, 2016). A helpful method that we can apply to any situation of working out what has happened and what to do about it is to ask the right sequence of questions, as identified in the following extract of a poem by Rudyard Kipling.

> *I keep six honest serving men*
> *(They taught me all I knew)*
> *Their names are What and Why and When*
> *And How and Where and Who.*
> (Kipling, 1902)

The five 'W' questions (Who/What/Where/When/Why) can be related to Chapters 1–3, while the 'H' question (How) is the main focus of clinical decision-making in this chapter, as follows.

Clinical judgement and decision-making in nursing

Who *does it involve?*   *Collaborative* (Chapter 2)

What *is the problem?*

Where *does it occur?*   *Observation* (Chapter 3)

When *does it occur?*

Why *make a decision?*   *Nursing theory* (Chapter 1)

How *to make decisions?*   *Systematic* (Chapter 4)

This relatively simple yet effective system of questions can be applied to reflect on situations we encounter and decisions we make in our professional development as nurses (Jasper et al., 2013). It can also help us to examine and integrate each stage of the decision-making process in nursing.

This chapter begins by clarifying what systematic clinical decision-making means, then explains and illustrates its use: (i) in a problem-solving nursing process; (ii) in addressing needs identified in the activities of living model; and (iii) in delivering sound, evidence-based, patient-centred care. Finally, the strengths and weaknesses of systematic clinical decision-making are summarised.

Activity 4.1 asks you to reflect on what was said in this chapter's introduction and then apply Kipling's questions to review a decision you have taken.

Activity 4.1   *Decision-making*

Given that the nurse's everyday decisions directly affect the lives of patients in their care, for the purposes of this activity try to identify and reflect on a decision you took regarding a significant event in your own life – for example, deciding to study nursing. Please apply Kipling's six questions to explore the decision-making process you went through. You might ask the following questions.

WHO?   Who did you consult before making a decision? Who else has been affected by it? Has the decision helped or hindered you in being who you want to be?

WHAT?   What made you commit three years of your life to study nursing? What might motivate or demotivate you to complete the programme?

WHERE?   Where did you live before and after starting the programme? Where else could you have studied? What made you opt to study nursing where you are now?

WHEN?   When you made your decision, what was happening in your life? What makes this the right time to study nursing?

WHY?   Why did you decide to study nursing? Why did you not choose other healthcare professions or non-health-related jobs?

HOW?   How did you hear about studying nursing? How did you prepare yourself for the selection interview? How have you adapted your lifestyle to be a student nurse?

After answering these questions in relation to a significant personal decision, write down how you think each of the six questions may help nurses to assess patients' health problems.

Some possible answers to the last question can be found at the end of the chapter.

Working through Activity 4.1 and applying the six questions to an event with which you are personally familiar should have helped you appreciate their potential usefulness in uncovering underlying factors that uniquely influence each judgement and decision in pursuing your life goals. Similarly, in applying the six questions to assess health problems, you have a practical tool to understand the unique way each individual patient experiences, and is affected by, ill health.

In order to relate this way of asking questions to nurses' systematic clinical decision-making, we need to find out more about the required skills and how to apply them.

What is systematic clinical decision-making?

Like other decision-making skills discussed in this book, systematic decisions were identified by researching nursing students' experience and understanding of their development in becoming registered nurses (Standing, 2005, 2007, 2010a). In the case study below, Jo, a nursing student, is asked to imagine that she is a patient and say what sort of nurse she would like to have.

Case study: Imagining oneself as a patient

Jo was asked about the qualities and skills she would value in a nurse if she was a patient (service user) needing care and attention. She replied:

'I want a nurse who is always thinking about what they are doing and why they are doing it. If I am prescribed medication, I don't want a nurse to simply give the drug because the doctor says so; I want a nurse who is going to think, "Why does this person need this drug? Is it the correct dose? In what form should it be given? When should it be given? What potential unwanted side effects from the drug may occur?" If I have to have an operation, I want a nurse who is going to think "Is that really the best dressing to put on the wound?" If I happen to have burnt both my hands, I don't want a nurse in such a hurry to feed me it feels like the food is being "shovelled" into my mouth; I want a nurse who engages with me and is considerate of my preferred way of eating and drinking.'

In the case study, Jo illustrates how asking Who/What/Where/When/Why/How questions can make a useful contribution to systematic clinical judgement and decision-making. This is characterised by combining critical thinking and problem-solving skills in giving patient-centred nursing care. For the purposes of this book the meaning of these terms is taken as follows.

Critical thinking – purposefully question the basis of own and others' assumptions, address gaps in knowledge, challenge illogical or unethical beliefs or practice, evaluate strength of available evidence, and be able to make a logical, evidence-based argument and defend it if challenged.

Problem solving – dissatisfaction with a current situation prompts use of critical thinking skills to identify and assess problem, plan and implement action to remedy it, and check if it worked.

Systematic clinical decisions – use of critical thinking and problem-solving skills to identify/assess patient's problem, set goals/make plans, deliver care and evaluate outcome (revise as needed).

In Table 4.1, Jo's use of critical thinking is related to Bloom's (1956) range of cognitive ability.

Level 1 (knowledge) is the simplest and level 6 (evaluation) is the most complex critical thinking skill in systematic decision-making. Knowledge and comprehension (levels 1–2) relate to theoretical understanding. Application and analysis (levels 3–4) are where theory is applied to practice in the delivery of nursing care. Synthesis and evaluation (levels 5–6) show a high degree of integration of theory and practice, each of which influences the other. Jo's examples (in which she alludes to the five 'Ws' and 'H' questions) relate to the whole range of critical thinking skills. Synthesis and evaluation are key graduate skills that are needed to enable nurses to make complex clinical judgements and decisions. Hence critical thinking skills are now seen as vital elements in effective problem solving and systematic clinical decision-making by nurses.

Level	Critical thinking	Jo's examples
1	Knowledge (remember things)	Know about – medication, its correct dose and purpose; types of wound dressings; care of burns; principles of feeding patients.
2	Comprehension (understand things)	Understand implications of knowledge, e.g. how medicine helps relieve patients' symptoms or why unwanted side effects occur.
3	Application (do things)	Use knowledge/understanding to assess needs and inform care.
4	Analysis (examine things)	Question plan of care and the roles and responsibilities of nurse, patient, doctor in its formulation and implementation.
5	Synthesis (create things)	Combine knowledge, skills, attitudes to ensure care has sound rationale, is technically competent, and is sensitively delivered (empathise with and help burns victim unable to feed himself).
6	Evaluation (critique things)	Review nursing interventions and outcomes of care and modify care plan if needed, e.g. use alternative wound dressing.

Table 4.1: Different levels of critical thinking skills in systematic decision-making

Activity 4.2 asks you to relate critical thinking to your own 'patient' view of nursing.

Activity 4.2   *Reflection and critical thinking*

Take a moment to reflect on Jo's view of nursing from a patient's perspective. Imagine you are a patient and write down what you would value about the qualities and skills of the nurses. Think of some examples and match them to the different levels of critical thinking in Table 4.1. Notice whether there are aspects of problem solving and systematic decision-making in your examples. You may want to compare notes with some of your colleagues to see how much you agree or disagree with each other.

As this is for your own reflection, no outline answer is given.

Activity 4.2 reminds us that combining critical thinking and problem-solving skills in systematic clinical decision-making is of little value unless it is patient-centred, effectively addressing the patient's needs and preferences. In the next section we look at how the nursing process revolutionised individualised systematic problem solving.

The nursing process and systematic decision-making

The nursing process was developed in the USA in the 1970s, applying scientific methods within a systematic and continuous cycle of problem solving, to guide individualised nursing care. In the early 1980s the introduction of the nursing process in the UK can be likened to the policy (and impact) of evidence-based practice in twenty-first-century healthcare. Both the nursing process and evidence-based practice offer a means to apply theory to practice in a logical, organised and systematic way to: (i) improve the quality of care; and (ii) effectively address patients' needs, health problems and preferences. Figure 4.1 identifies the key stages in the nursing process, summarises their specific function in problem solving and illustrates the process's ongoing cyclical nature (adapted from an original description by Yura and Walsh, 1973). As such, it provides a useful structure with which to understand and apply the principles of systematic clinical decision-making in nursing.

- Assessment (and reassessment) of patients' health problems and care needs

- Planning strategies to address the identified health problems and care needs

- Implementing agreed nursing interventions in delivering individualised care

- Evaluation of care outcomes to see if problems have been resolved or not

Figure 4.1: Nursing process

The stages shown in Figure 4.1 broadly correspond to Peplau's theory of interpersonal relations in mental health nursing (Chapter 1), but with more emphasis on problem solving and less on relationship building. In addition, the nursing process can be applied in any field of healthcare.

This process represents a very significant development in the professional identity of nurses, as it provided us with the tools to independently and systematically assess patients' needs and plan, deliver and evaluate care. Applying the nursing process effectively enables nurses to be autonomous health professionals. The case study below illustrates systematic clinical decision-making using Who/What/Where/When/Why/How questions within the nursing process.

Case study: Using who, what, where, when, why and how questions

Michelle, a second-year student on placement in a children's hospital unit, is asked by her mentor to admit Ann and her three-month-old son Eric, and carry out an assessment. Michelle uses the five 'Ws' and 'H' questions (who has a problem, what it is, where and when it is, and why and how it is a problem) when asking Ann to explain her concerns about Eric.

WHO?   *Eric has a feeding problem and Ann has become sore from breastfeeding him.*

WHAT?   *Eric is vomiting after feeding, he always seems hungry and he is not gaining weight.*

WHERE?   *Usually at home but also when visiting family – anywhere, in fact, if he has had a feed.*

WHEN?   *Soon after feeding. It has been getting progressively worse over the last few weeks.*

WHY?   *Ann has breastfed Eric, so she tried baby formula bottle milk instead to see if it made a difference, but it did not. She even tried different brands of baby milk, but Eric continued to vomit. She is worried that Eric is not going to survive if something is not done to keep his feed down.*

HOW?   *Sometimes it is 'like a white fountain shooting out of his mouth' (projectile vomiting), and after being sick Eric wants to feed again straightaway. Michelle asks Ann if she can watch the next time she feeds Eric. Ann breastfeeds Eric, and shortly after he vomits back the milk.*

Michelle discusses the assessment with her mentor, who asks her to accompany Ann and Eric to radiology for an ultrasound examination of Eric's stomach. The results show he has pyloric stenosis (narrowing of the passage between the stomach and small intestine caused by build-up of muscle) preventing sufficient food from being absorbed. The medical diagnosis explains Eric's symptoms and he is scheduled for keyhole surgery (laparoscopic pyloromyotomy) the next day to remove excess muscle. The nursing care plan includes pre- and post-operative care of Eric, monitoring the intravenous line (inserted by a doctor) and fluids, checking and cleaning the wound near his belly button and reintroducing milk feeds the day after surgery. Michelle also asks her mentor if she can give Ann some Vaseline to heal sores before she breastfeeds again as she was so concerned about Eric that she forgot to bring some for herself. Ann is relieved that they know what the problem is, that she is not to blame in any way and was right to seek help, and that the operation usually completely cures the problem. She also appreciates Michelle's concern for her. A day after surgery Eric feeds without vomiting and the next day Ann takes him home.

Eric's condition required surgical intervention to cure it, but resolving his problem also depended on the nursing care he and his mother received. By applying the five 'Ws' and 'H' questions in the assessment, Michelle gained an understanding of not only the main health problem (Eric vomits after feeding) but also how it was affecting both Eric (always hungry, not gaining weight) and Ann (fearful about Eric dying, anxious to know what the problem is, feeling guilty that she might be at fault, and sore from breastfeeding a baby who is never satisfied). Hence, care delivery depended on collaboration (Chapter 2) and observation (Chapter 3) as nurses complemented the surgical team by controlling: (i) pre-operative risks (ensure Eric is clean, well hydrated from intravenous fluids, nil by mouth so stomach empty to prevent inhalation of vomit during surgery); and (ii) post-operative risks (risk of post-anaesthetic vomiting, ensure airway kept clear, prevent infection of wound and intravenous line). The nurses also collaborated closely with Ann in enabling her to understand what was wrong with Eric, being supportive in understanding her concerns and helping to relieve her soreness. This was necessary for Ann to be physically and psychologically refreshed and ready to care for Eric, including gradually resuming feeding him the day after his operation. This helped to ensure that the most important collaborative relationship – bonding between mother and baby – was enhanced by the experience they shared in hospital, which was vital for Eric's future healthy development.

The case study shows how the nursing process can guide nurses' systematic clinical judgement and decision-making in assessment, planning, delivery and evaluation of care. It also illustrates how using the nursing process enables us to complement the roles of other health professionals (e.g. the surgical team) while ensuring care is tailored to the individual needs of patients and their families. Our chances of success in achieving both these aims is increased by continually using the five 'Ws' and 'H' questions to identify and review not just health problems but also how they affect the individuals concerned. Questioning develops our critical thinking (know, understand, do, examine, create and critique), which helps us to integrate problem-solving and patient-centred care in systematic clinical judgement and decision-making. Activity 4.3 asks you to use your critical thinking skills to review how the nursing process is applied in practice.

Activity 4.3   *Decision-making and critical thinking*

Each clinical practice setting often looks after patients with similar healthcare problems, which can result in similarities in the systematic assessment, planning and delivery of nursing care. The aim of this activity is for you to compare and contrast care plans for patients with similar conditions in order to see whether there is any variation in the care plans, and if they do vary, whether it reflects patients' different individual circumstances or some other reason. If care is truly patient-centred, we would expect some variation in care plans, and if there is little difference between them, it suggests they could be tailored better to each patient's unique situation. Suppose your mentor asks you to propose a way of making the care plans more patient-centred. What strategies can you suggest for making nursing care plans more relevant and responsive to patients' individual differences?

Some possible answers can be found at the end of the chapter.

Activity 4.3 assumes you will find that the nursing process is still widely used in clinical practice to guide the systematic assessment, planning, delivery and evaluation of care. The process also encourages nurses to keep accurate records, which aids communication in the healthcare team and provides evidence of clinical judgements, decisions and actions – for which they are accountable.

The continuing relevance of the nursing process in twenty-first-century nursing is evident by its inclusion in the *Standards for pre-registration nursing education* (NMC, 2010) shown at the start of this chapter, and in the International Council of Nurses competency framework for post-registration specialist nurses (ICN, 2009).

Some have criticised the focus on problem solving in the nursing process as being too much like a medical model and not capturing the uniqueness of nursing (Parse, 1992), or so standardised that individualised care is overlooked (Benner, 1984). Others argue that the nursing process ought to be supplemented by critical thinking skills (Corcoran-Perry and Narayan, 1995; Alfaro-LeFevre, 2013), and used in tandem with more comprehensive nursing theories/models (Griffith and Christensen, 1982). In completing Activity 4.3, you were faced with some of these issues and asked to work out a solution. In the next section we explore how combining the nursing process with the activities of a living model can help relate theory to practice in individualising systematic clinical decision-making.

Activities of living and systematic decision-making

In the previous case study we saw how the nursing process guides systematic decision-making in identifying a problem and contributing to its resolution (Eric's digestion of food and fluids was compromised by an abnormality in his stomach requiring surgical correction). Eating and drinking is one of 12 activities of living described by Roper et al. (2000) that we engage in to satisfy physical, psychological and social needs (see Table 4.2, left-hand column). Activities of living, prioritised in caring for Eric, were: breathing (risk of inhaling vomit); maintaining safe environment (unable to protect himself); and personal cleansing and dressing (risk of infection). The 'activities of living' model is therefore helpful in directing our attention to problems patients may have, and in understanding *why* this threatens their health and wellbeing. It is a valuable theoretical framework to combine with the nursing process in applying systematic clinical decision-making in individualised, patient-centred care. Table 4.2 applies the concepts of *human being, environment, health* and *nurse's role and decision-making* used in Chapter 1 (Table 1.1) to the activities of living model. Each activity of living is influenced by physical, psychological, 'sociocultural' (including spiritual), environmental and 'politicoeconomic' (including legal) factors. Furthermore, a person's ability to carry out these activities varies from complete independence to complete dependence upon others in relation to health status, stage of development in lifespan and individual choice.

The 12 activities of living listed in Table 4.2 apply to all of us as human beings, and the way we carry them out is affected by environmental factors and our individual (physical and psychological) differences and preferences. The model offers us, as nurses, a comprehensive and practical guide to understanding each patient as a unique individual while identifying activities of living they are having problems with that require our help. It incorporates the nursing process to guide our systematic clinical judgement and decision-making in individualised care according to problems identified during assessment and the priorities and goals of the resulting care plans. In this way the model helps us to look beyond a medical condition or illness and gain a more holistic understanding of how health problems impact on individual patients and their families.

Human being	Environment	Health	Nurse's role and decision-making
Have bio-psycho-social-spiritual needs individually met via activities of living: Maintaining a safe environment Communicating Breathing Eating and drinking Eliminating Cleansing and dressing Controlling body temperature Mobilising Working and playing Expressing sexuality Sleeping Dying	*Physical:* source of air, water, food, warmth, shelter, modes of transport *Sociocultural:* roles, relationships and ethical or spiritual beliefs and values shaped by culture *Politicoeconomic:* legislation controls the distribution of healthcare funding and resources	*Health:* associated with independence of individuals in carrying out their activities of living during lifespan as befits their age (dependent baby is usually healthy) *Ill health:* physical or psychological, associated with more dependence on others in one's activities of living	Give individualised, systematic care by: collaborating with patients (and others) to *assess* their level of independence and dependence in the activities of living; setting goals, *planning* care to complement and/or supplementing patients' ability to carry out activities of living; *implementing* interventions; and, *evaluating* outcomes.

Table 4.2: Activities of living model (Roper et al., 2000) and systematic decision-making

Some of the activities of living, such as breathing or eating and drinking, appear to have more immediate relevance to our health and sense of wellbeing. The relevance of others, such as communicating, may be less obvious, but the case study illustrated the importance of communicating as Eric was unable to tell anyone what was wrong with him, and without his mother advocating on his behalf he would not have received vital medical and nursing care. 'Expressing sexuality' may, at first glance, seem a strange one to consider in a nursing assessment, but we cannot treat people as individuals without acknowledging their sexuality, and in some situations this is related to specific health problems. Even Eric's medical problem (infantile pyloric stenosis) is gender related as boys are four times more susceptible than girls (Hernanz-Schulman, 2003). Similarly, 'dying' is not something that immediately springs to mind when thinking about what we do every day, but we know it is inevitable, and illness, accident or conflict can threaten survival at any time. In the case study, Ann's fear that Eric could die was understandable (although mortality rates are now low for pyloric stenosis). Originally the condition was identified only by post-mortem examination, and around 100 years ago 50 per cent of babies with the condition died from it (Hernanz-Schulman, 2003).

The next case study applies the activities of living model to systematic decision-making with an adult patient who has a long-term medical condition for which there is no known cure.

Case study: Assessing a patient's activities of living

Serena is a student nurse at the end of her second year on placement in a medical unit. During 'handover' she hears about Charlotte, aged 47, a new admission with a medical diagnosis of multiple sclerosis (erosion of the protective insulation 'myelin sheath' around the nerves) with a history of remissions, when she is fairly independent, and relapses, when she is highly dependent. Over the last two years the relapses have become more frequent and severe. On this occasion her partner Anita raised the alarm because she can no longer physically cope. Serena is asked by her mentor to apply the activities of living model to assess Charlotte's problems, set goals and plan care.

Maintaining a safe environment Problem: *Charlotte cannot stand or walk unassisted, has poor hand co-ordination, poor eyesight and lacks feeling in hands and feet.* Goal: *prevent injury from falling, having accident or scalding herself.* Plan: *closely observe/supervise all activities, review ways to lengthen remission periods with medical team, e.g. treatment to boost immune system.*

Communicating Problem: *Charlotte has difficulty in speaking clearly.* Goal: *to understand what Charlotte's likes and dislikes are, and help her express herself.* Plan: *allow more time for her to talk, observe body language, refer for speech and language therapy (SALT) assessment and ask Anita for communication tips.*

Breathing Problem: *when Charlotte's saliva goes down the wrong way she has coughing fit.* Goal: *prevent choking and chest infection.* Plan: *when awake support Charlotte in sitting up so she can take deep breaths, and when asleep turn her onto her side to keep her airway clear.*

Eating and drinking Problem: *Charlotte has difficulty in swallowing.* Goal: *ensure adequate and safe (avoid choking) fluids and nutrition.* Plan: *fluid chart, minimum 2 litres daily, check weight, refer to dietitian and SALT team, give non-spill easy-to-hold cup, assist Charlotte to feed herself.*

Eliminating Problem: *Charlotte has poor bladder control, smelly urine and constipation.* Goal: *prevent urinary incontinence and infection, and relieve constipation.* Plan: *send urine sample for analysis, record output on fluid chart, two-hourly toileting, high-fibre supplements and laxatives.*

Personal cleansing/dressing Problem: *Charlotte cannot bathe herself, and dresses/undresses with difficulty.* Goal: *good personal hygiene and well attired.* Plan: *enable Charlotte to wash hands/face, give daily 'sit in' bath/shower and ask Anita to bring loose, comfortable clothes.*

Controlling body temperature Problem: *Charlotte's hands and feet are often cold to touch.* Goal: *prevent hands and feet from getting cold.* Plan: *ask Anita for warm socks and mittens, encourage Charlotte to wriggle toes and rub hands together, and inform medical team about it.*

(Continued)

---

continued . . .

Mobilising Problem: *Charlotte is immobile, has spasms and stiffness in legs; skin lacks elasticity and she is at risk of getting pressure sores.* Goal: *prevent pressure sores and muscle wasting, and relieve stiffness.* Plan: *assess and monitor pressure area risks using Waterlow scale, provide pressure relief mattress/seat cushion, change position every two hours, encourage passive limb movement, refer to physiotherapy, give prescribed medication (corticosteroids), ask medical team about research supporting use of cannabis to treat spasms/stiffness, use approved lifting techniques and equipment (slide sheets, hoist) and co-ordinate teamwork to change her position or move her from bed to chair safely (without scraping her skin, alarming her or injuring nurses).*

Working and playing Problem: *when in remission Charlotte volunteers in a charity shop; she used to enjoy reading before sight deteriorated and she likes classical music.* Goal: *enable Charlotte to experience things that she enjoys.* Plan: *check with medical team whether sight can be improved, check library service for talking books or music she might like to listen to.*

Expressing sexuality Problem: *Charlotte is upset by physical deterioration and feels unattractive.* Goal: *support Charlotte in recognising her attractive qualities.* Plan: *acknowledge Charlotte's achievements in doing what she can for herself, refer to beautician to manicure nails, encourage her to comb or brush hair before Anita visits and make positive remarks about her appearance.*

Sleeping Problem: *Charlotte's sleep could be disturbed due to her being turned regularly.* Goal: *minimise sleep disturbance when turning her.* Plan: *explain nurses will carefully turn her from side to side every two hours and why it is important (so she is not taken too much by surprise if she wakes up), and ask Charlotte if she would like the doctor to prescribe sleeping tablets.*

Dying Problem: *Charlotte is frightened about dying.* Goal: *give Charlotte accurate information about her illness, treatment and expected outcomes in a supportive manner.* Plan: *ask doctor to explain Charlotte's prognosis regarding her current relapse and future life expectancy; ask Charlotte if she would like Anita to be present when the doctor talks to her and ensure that Charlotte and Anita have details of the Multiple Sclerosis Society where they can get more information and support.*

The case study illustrates how the activities of living model complements the nursing process in directing systematic clinical judgement and decision-making in comprehensive assessment and care planning. The focus on activities of living helps us to recognise that our role complements and supplements patients' own abilities and their level of dependence or independence. It offers an accessible structure to address a wide range of bio-psycho-social-spiritual health issues specifically tailored to each patient's unique circumstances. It also indicates how complex nursing decisions can be, while reinforcing the value of observation and collaboration with patients, families/carers and the inter-professional healthcare team. Activity 4.4 asks you to apply the activities of living model to your own clinical practice before we look at systematic clinical decision-making in evidence-based practice.

Practise applying the 12 activities of living in Table 4.2 (examples are given in the case study), and apply them to systematically assess problems, set goals and plan care for patients you have cared for in the past or you are currently caring for. Discuss your care plan with your mentor.

As this is for you to consolidate learning in relating it to your experience, there is no outline answer.

Systematic clinical decision-making in patient-centred evidence-based practice

The case studies we have looked at so far are forms of evidence because they are based on real people, events and nursing interventions that have been examined and discussed by applying relevant theory and research. In the final case study we go one step further in enabling service users to apply critical thinking and problem-solving skills using a well-researched therapy. The patient is the 'primary practitioner' in highly systematic, evidence-based self-care, while the nurse adopts a collaborative, educative and supportive role. We are going to be looking at the application of cognitive behaviour therapy (CBT) by someone with anxiety and panic attacks. It is the method of choice for the treatment of anxiety in the National Institute for Health and Care Excellence clinical guidelines (NICE, 2011). Beck (2011) summarises the main principles of CBT as follows.

1. Emotions and related behaviour are prompted by our beliefs.
2. Distorted perceptions and false beliefs can cause emotional problems.
3. Correcting inaccurate, self-defeating beliefs can resolve emotional problems.

Applying CBT principles in service users' self-care

Teach service users to treat themselves by being able to:

A monitor their emotional responses and behaviour;

B identify trigger events associated with A;

C identify related unhelpful beliefs and thoughts;

D make connections between thinking, emotions and behaviour;

E examine evidence for and against unhelpful beliefs;

F replace unhelpful thoughts with realistic helpful thoughts.
(Adapted from Trower et al., 1988)

The following case study shows how a nurse therapist is teaching a client to apply CBT to help her deal with her anxiety and panic attacks. She has set the client homework in using an ABC framework (Ellis and Dryden, 2007) where A = activating event associated with anxiety, B = beliefs about the event (differentiate between helpful and unhelpful thoughts and images) and C = consequences of beliefs about the events (differentiate between helpful and unhelpful emotions and behaviour). The aim is to empower the client to recognise how her overly negative self-critical thoughts can make her feel bad, and to replace these with self-affirming thoughts that accurately reflect evidence of her positive characteristics (not usually acknowledged) in order for her to feel less anxious.

Case study: Self-care using CBT to challenge self-denigrating beliefs

Kim is a third-year student on placement in a community mental health team. She accompanies one of the nurses, Rita, a qualified cognitive behaviour therapist, to visit Carol, aged 34, referred by her GP as she gets panic attacks and is frightened of going out. Carol was divorced seven years ago, lives with daughter Judy, aged 11, and works as an assistant librarian. Last month she had to take Judy to visit her new school. Carol was very nervous about going, and when she got there had a severe panic attack (heart thumping, sweaty, dizzy, felt sick and was desperate for the toilet). Since then she feels safe only when at home, has had time off work, will not go shopping unless Judy is with her and is very reluctant to go out anywhere. Rita saw Carol twice last week to do an initial assessment, explain how Carol could apply CBT to deal with problems, explore what happened, how she felt and what was on her mind at the school.

Rita begins by checking that Carol remembers her saying she would have a student this week and explains Kim is there to observe. She asks Carol how she feels about this. Carol says it is not a problem and she is happy for Kim to observe. Rita asks Carol if she can apply CBT to look at her decision-making in her acceptance of Kim. Carol responds by getting out one of the blank 'ABC' forms Rita gave her, and puts 'happy for Kim to observe' under C (consequences) – helpful emotions/behaviours. She puts 'Kim turning up with Rita' under A (activating event). Rita confirms that Carol correctly identified the event that triggered her decision-making and the outcome. She is aware that Carol has not identified her beliefs and asks Carol if the event itself was sufficient to bring about the outcome or if something else was needed. Carol says she knows she has to put something under B but cannot think what it is. Rita asks Carol again to at look at whether A is sufficient to explain C and she says, 'Well, we all have to learn, don't we? I remember having to shadow the librarian.' 'Ah,' Rita says. 'I think you have just identified a belief about A.' Carol writes 'We all have to learn' under B (beliefs) – helpful thoughts/images. Rita asks Carol if there is anything about Kim's behaviour that might have contributed to her decision, and she says, 'Well, she seems to be taking it all in and is used to seeing mad people like me.' Rita suggests Carol puts the first part of her answer under B (beliefs) – helpful thoughts/ images – and asks her where she thinks the second part ('she is used to seeing mad people like me') should go. Carol pauses then puts it under B (beliefs) – unhelpful thoughts/images. Rita asks Carol to read out the completed ABC form and explain it to Kim. Carol tells Kim it helps her to understand that it is how she makes sense of events that determines how she feels or behaves, rather than the events themselves, so she is more in control and also has an opportunity to change from unhelpful to helpful beliefs, which makes her feel more confident.

Table 4.3 is a summary of this brief exchange in the ABC format Carol has learnt to apply to herself.

continued . . .

'A' Activating event (describe an experience)	'B' Beliefs (about A) (your thoughts/images)	'C' Consequences (of 'B') (your emotions/behaviour)
Rita (nurse therapist) arrives with Kim (nursing student)	*Helpful:* we all have to learn; it is like when I had to shadow the librarian at work. She (Kim) seems to be 'taking it all in'. *Unhelpful:* Kim is used to seeing mad people like me.	*Helpful:* It is not a problem. I am happy for Kim to observe. I feel I am doing something useful in helping Kim to learn. *Unhelpful:* self 'put down' 'takes the shine off' my efforts to feel more self-confident.

Table 4.3: Carol's self-completed 'ABC' form applying CBT

Rita points out that Carol's beliefs in this instance concern Kim, and she has a golden opportunity to test the evidence (her assumptions about Kim) by checking with Kim. Kim agrees she is there to learn, that she has learnt stuff she did not know before from both of them and that she does not think Carol is mad. Rita suggests that Kim has played her part in supporting the evidence for Carol's helpful beliefs while helping her to challenge her unhelpful beliefs, and although Carol may have said it in jest, it revealed her self-denigration, and the consequences of it can add to her anxiety, panic attacks and fear of going out. Rita sets Carol homework to complete an 'ABC' form focusing on her fear of going to the surgery, which she will explore with her next time.

The case study shows how evidence-based CBT can be applied in community mental healthcare. It complements observation of physical factors, mood, thoughts and behaviour in assessing mental health (Chapter 3), and the Who/What/Where/When/Why/How questions discussed earlier. The nurse therapist was skilful in enabling the client to apply CBT to explore her reaction to the nursing student observing her, a potentially anxiety-inducing event. The student also made a positive contribution by giving feedback about the accuracies and inaccuracies of the client's assumptions about her. This provided evidence to support Carol's helpful, realistic beliefs while challenging her unhelpful, unrealistic beliefs. She also seemed to gain confidence in using the 'ABC' structure for self-assessment. Table 4.4 relates Rita and Kim's systematic decision-making (in enabling Carol's self-care using CBT) to the conceptions of nursing.

In the case study the use of CBT helped the patient to become aware of judgements and decisions she had made about herself that contributed to her feeling anxious, having panic attacks and avoiding going out. It gave her the tools to test evidence that challenged her negative view of herself and enabled her to work towards a more realistic self-appraisal. This in turn will give her a greater sense of control and self-confidence to overcome her anxieties as she gradually learns to venture out again. While this case study relates to mental health, it applies the principles of person-centred, evidence-based, systematic decision-making relevant to all fields of nursing. Activity 4.5 asks you to test out CBT techniques in relation to your own experience.

Conceptions of nursing	Systematic clinical decision-making
Caring	Support and validate Carol's ability to help herself.
Listening and being there	Be alert to negative beliefs Carol expresses about herself.
Practical procedures	Conduct interview, set new homework, arrange next visit.
Knowledge and understanding	Use principles of CBT for anxiety/panic attacks/low self-esteem.
Communicating	Question Carol about thoughts/feelings, use of CBT; give feedback to support helpful/challenge unhelpful thoughts.
Patience	Give Carol time to categorise and record thoughts/feelings.
Teamwork	Kim complemented Rita by helping Carol test assumptions.
Paperwork and electronic record	Give Carol 'ABC' forms so she can examine and record events, beliefs triggered by them and how they affect her.
Empathising and non-judgemental	Understand Carol might be anxious about Kim's presence.
Professional	Apply evidence-based, NICE approved, CBT interventions.

Table 4.4: Integrating systematic clinical decision-making with conceptions of nursing

Activity 4.5   *Evidence-based practice and research*

Use the 'ABC' framework shown in Table 4.5.

(i)   Identify an emotional experience you have had and describe the event under A.

(ii) Describe how this made you feel (e.g. anxious/sad/angry) and behave under 'C'.

(iii) Now try to fill in the gap regarding your personal interpretation of the event under 'B', i.e. what it 'says about you', why you think this is true and how these beliefs (rather than the event itself) may have left you feeling the way you did.

(iv) Try to separate helpful from unhelpful beliefs and consequences.

(v)   Review the evidence for and against your beliefs.

(vi) Reflect on how some beliefs might be based on false assumptions and use this awareness to challenge overly negative, self-defeating internal dialogue with evidence to the contrary.

'A' Activating event (describe an experience)	'B' Beliefs (about A) (your thoughts/images)	'C' Consequences (of 'B') (your emotions/behaviour)
	Helpful:	Helpful:
	Unhelpful:	Unhelpful:

Table 4.5: The 'ABC' framework

As this activity is for your own personal research there is no answer provided, but self-help books applying CBT techniques can be found in the further reading section.

Activity 4.5 can help us to understand how events can trigger thoughts that determine how we feel and behave. This is important because unless we are able to separate and examine these different elements, we might remain unaware of our reasoning behind decisions – and our beliefs may be mistaken. The use of CBT to examine how well our decisions match up to the available evidence encourages us to be more aware of our own biases and 'blind spots' (see also reflexivity in Chapter 8). It also complements critical thinking ability, which is a vital aspect of effective systematic clinical decision-making. In Chapter 5 we will look in more detail at evidence-based practice in relation to standardised policies, procedures and clinical guidelines.

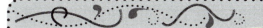

Chapter summary

This chapter defined and explored systematic clinical decision-making in relation to asking Who/What/Where/When/Why/How questions, enabling nurses to apply critical thinking and problem solving with patients to address their needs. We incorporated this questioning approach in applying the nursing process, an influential framework supporting systematic clinical decision-making. The strengths of systematic clinical decision-making are that it enables patient assessment and problem solving to ensure the planning and delivery of care is relevant to their needs. It also promotes nurses' use of critical thinking skills in continually evaluating the effectiveness of interventions to give patients high quality care. The weaknesses of systematic clinical decision-making are that patients may be seen as health problems rather than people, and this can detract from truly patient-centred nursing care. We saw that the nursing process needs to be supplemented by theory and research to guide more comprehensive, patient-centred assessment/care planning, and the 'activities of living' model was shown to marry very well with it. We then supplemented the nursing process with cognitive behaviour therapy (CBT) techniques in teaching mental health patients how they can apply systematic decision-making to their self-care. We explored how using CBT techniques encourages service users/patients to learn how to question the basis of their own assumptions, especially where this leads to emotional or behavioural problems. We saw how changes could be made by raising awareness of self-defeating 'internal dialogue', and challenging overly negative and unrealistic belief systems with contrary evidence. This offers great potential in empowering service users, but also in enabling nurses to be self-aware and apply critical thinking skills in systematic clinical decision-making.

Activities: brief outline answers

Activity 4.1: Decision-making (page 59)

You may have included some of the following points.

WHO?   Who is the patient? Who are their significant others? If infectious, who have they had contact with? Who else needs to be involved in their care?

WHAT?   What has made the patient seek help? What aspects of their bio-psycho-social-spiritual needs do they have difficulty with? What are their most urgent needs?

WHERE?   If in pain, where does it hurt? If in an accident, where did it happen? If a psychological problem, which social or environmental settings make it better or worse?

WHEN?	When did they first notice the problem? When does it affect them? During year/month/day/night? When doing certain activities? Are they experiencing the problem now?
WHY?	Why does the patient think they developed a health problem? Why are they unable to resolve it themselves? Why is nursing care needed (or not) for the patient?
HOW?	How has the patient's life been affected by the problem? How have they/their families/others managed to cope with it so far? How can nursing care make a difference?

Activity 4.3: Decision-making and critical thinking (page 64)

You may have included some of the following points.

- Incorporate Who/What/Where/When/Why/How questions, especially when assessing/reassessing patients (see answer guide to Activity 4.1).

- As well as identifying the health problem, find out how it is affecting the patient and family, and use this knowledge to inform individualised aspects of the care plan.

- Combine systematic/collaborative/observation in decision-making so patients' needs and preferences influence care plans, which are continually evaluated and revised as needed.

- Review patients' care plans using Bloom's range of critical thinking skills (see Table 4.1) to explore ways of making them more relevant to each patient's needs.

Further reading

Ellis, P (2016) *Evidence-based practice in nursing* (3rd edn). London: Sage/Learning Matters.

Excellent introduction to evidence-based practice for nurses applying many different types of evidence.

Holland, K, Jenkins, J, Solomon, J and Whittam, S (2008) *Applying the Roper-Logan-Tierney model in practice.* Edinburgh: Churchill Livingstone.

Case studies of activities of living model guiding evidence-based problem solving.

Howatson-Jones, L, Standing, M and Roberts, S (2015) *Patient assessment and care planning in nursing* (2nd edn). London: Sage/Learning Matters.

Applies critical thinking skills to patient assessment and care in hospital/community settings.

Kennerley, H (2014) *Overcoming anxiety* (2nd edn). London: Constable & Robinson.

A valuable self-help guide enabling users to apply cognitive behaviour therapy (CBT) techniques to manage their anxieties.

Silove, D and Manicavasgar, V (2009) *Overcoming panic and agoraphobia.* London: Constable & Robinson.

A valuable self-help guide enabling users to apply CBT techniques to control panic feelings and/or fear of going out.

Useful websites

www.mssociety.org.uk

Award-winning Multiple Sclerosis Society website packed with the latest information, research and advice for patients, carers and professionals.

www.rebt.ws/REBT%20explained.htm

The 'ABC' framework adopted in the last case study is explained in more depth by Dr Albert Ellis, the founder of rational emotive behaviour therapy/REBT (a form of CBT).

Chapter 5
Standardised clinical decision-making

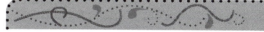

Introduction

At the start of each chapter in this book (and other books in the same series) you see selected NMC *Standards for pre-registration nursing education* (2010) and related competencies. These are examples of standardisation, which involves identifying minimum acceptable standards for any product or process and then ensuring that all examples conform to the agreed formula. Setting standards in nursing education helps prepare you in the knowledge, skills, attitudes, values and standards of professional conduct (NMC, 2015) that you need to demonstrate as a registered nurse.

Standardisation is prevalent in all walks of life; for example, you could go into any restaurant of a particular fast food chain anywhere in the world and expect to get the same meal prepared to the same standard. The formula is successful because the product is popular and keenly priced, and customers know what to expect. Getting it right requires ongoing market research to develop appealing recipes, policies and business plans and to update them as required. This ensures the effective management of restaurants in sourcing, preparing and serving flavoursome meals, responding to new developments (e.g. sugar-free alternatives to high-sugar soft drinks) and satisfying customers. The same basic principles are applied in assuring the quality of good-value healthcare, which is also influenced by research evidence, national policies, standards and guidelines, responding to new developments (e.g. growth of antibiotic-resistant bacteria has prompted doctors to consider alternatives to prescribing them) and feedback from service users. Hence, healthcare professionals are required to follow agreed clinical procedures to ensure that care or treatment is safe and effective, with a high level of patient satisfaction.

In this chapter we apply the principles of standardisation to clinical decision-making in nursing. We start by clarifying what standardisation means and then look at its application in local clinical procedures and the influence of government health policy and evidence-based clinical guidelines. Finally, the strengths and weaknesses of **standardised clinical decision-making** are summarised.

What is standardised clinical decision-making?

Standardised clinical decision-making was identified as a significant theme when researching nursing students' perceptions, experience and development of clinical decision-making skills (Standing, 2005, 2007, 2010a), as illustrated in the following case study.

Case study: Students' perceptions of standardised decision-making

After 18 months on a pre-registration nursing programme, students were asked to describe their experience and involvement in patient care and how they perceived clinical decision-making. A number of them made similar comments about the apparent predetermined or prescribed nature of many nursing decisions, particularly in relation to assessment and planning care.

Some students saw standardised decision-making as a positive thing.

- *'Luckily they use Roper's model, which I am keen on. The care plans and assessment forms are all preprinted so you just follow a list of questions.'*
- *'The care plans are computerised and they have highly structured forms to fill in so that you cannot forget to ask about things that are relevant.'*
- *'The standardised care plans on the ward very much cover all the angles. So care planning is "covering all the bases" making sure you have an appropriate response for almost anything that might happen.'*

Other students were less enthusiastic about standardised decision-making.

- *'Every ward has a filing cabinet full of core care plans.'*
- *'You get a patient, you go to a drawer, and there is a numbered care plan.'*
- *'We use core care plans following the Roper model but I don't like them.'*

The case study suggests that the nursing process and activities of living model (Roper et al., 2000) – discussed in relation to systematic decision-making in Chapter 4 – were adopted as standardised templates to assess patients' problems or needs, and in planning care. Students who thought this was a good thing appreciated the way it helped them know what to ask patients, how to record their responses and how this contributes to the delivery of effective patient care. For other students standardised 'core care plans' appeared part of a task-orientated routine in which they were unable to identify any specific benefits either for patients or for themselves. To optimise the benefits of standardised decision-making (e.g. not having to 'reinvent the wheel' in care plans for patients with similar problems) we need to combine it with observation, collaborative and systematic decision-making (Chapters 2–4), so that care meets patients' individual needs.

In some cases the core care plans referred to by students were not restricted to nursing as they represented the total care received by patients from all of the healthcare professionals concerned. These are examples of integrated care pathways (ICPs) that are characterised by the following features.

- Use standardised, systematic, collaborative and inter-professional care planning.
- Focus on patients who share a similar medical condition or health problem.
- Are developed, implemented and audited locally by health professionals and patients.
- Incorporate latest relevant research findings to guide evidence-based practice.
- Identify key goals on the 'patient journey' from initial assessment to discharge.
- Co-ordinate roles and responsibilities for care by different healthcare professionals.
- Share inter-professional documenting of care, which avoids unnecessary duplication.
- Record variation from ICP goals and explain professional judgement.
- Give patients an outline of what to expect and how they can contribute to care.
- Enhance quality of care, reducing variations in standards among practitioners.

(Campbell et al., 1998; Middleton et al., 2001)

The complexity of health problems results in many different health and other professionals contributing to patients' treatment and care. Integrated care pathways are a useful way of co-ordinating and standardising clinical decision-making in the assessment, planning, delivery and evaluation of multidisciplinary health and social care. They enhance inter-professional communication and teamwork in delivering evidence-based care of a consistently high standard. Standardised clinical decision-making is influenced by many factors, including the nature of patients' problems, health policy, research, evidence-based clinical guidelines, local procedures, teamwork and the organisation of services (clinical governance). For the purposes of this book standardised clinical decision-making is defined as follows:

> *Standardised clinical decision-making applies NHS Trust policies and procedures, agreed care plans and evidence-based guidelines/assessment tools uniformly and consistently to patient care.*

Standardised clinical decision-making in nursing was identified by students reflecting on their experiences.

Activity 5.1   *Reflection*

How does your experience compare with that of students in the case study? Take a moment to think about your observations of standardised clinical decision-making regarding assessment tools, planning care, administering medication, clinical procedures and guidelines applied in your practice placements. Describe an example of standardised

continued . . .

decision-making; identify the intended benefits for patients, what the outcomes were, and what you learnt about clinical decision-making. Was your example of standardised decision-making supplemented by observation, collaborative decision-making or systematic decision-making? If so, how? Why do you think this was necessary? What was the effect of doing so?

As this is for your own reflection there is no outline answer provided.

Standardised decision-making in clinical procedures

So far we have ascertained that nursing education is standardised so that patients can receive safe, effective and competent care relevant to their needs, whichever registered nurse is on duty. We have looked at ways in which nurses' decision-making is standardised and how this may be complemented by observation, collaborative and systematic decision-making in tailoring care for each patient. The next case study combines these elements, as a student has to demonstrate competence in a clinical procedure to pass an assessment while also being sensitive to the patient's needs.

Case study: Catheterising complications

Lawrence is a registered mental health nurse doing a shortened post-registration adult nursing programme. He is on placement in an acute medical hospital ward where he is due to be assessed in carrying out a clinical procedure safely and effectively using aseptic 'non-touch' technique to avoid contaminating sterile areas. Lawrence is anxious because he is more skilled in talking to patients than he is in physical care but must pass to stay on the programme.

Frank, aged 68, a retired bricklayer, usually very fit, is admitted for investigations into why he has been tired over the last few weeks and unable to do gardening, which he normally loves, and why he has lower back pain. Frank cannot provide a urine sample, and medical examination reveals a distended bladder from chronic urinary retention associated with an enlarged prostate gland. Frank has not told anyone he has problems urinating before. Lawrence discusses Frank's care with his mentor. The goal is for Frank to empty his bladder. The plan is to catheterise Frank. Lawrence has observed and assisted in the procedure before and agrees to be assessed by his clinical mentor in catheterising Frank. He checks the clinical procedures manual. He asks Frank if he remembers what the doctor said about his bladder problem and he replies, 'I got a blocked pipe and need a plumber!' Lawrence explains urethral catheterisation and that anaesthetic gel will be used to reduce his discomfort, and he checks that Frank agrees to him carrying out the procedure with the mentor observing, which he does. Lawrence says he will be

(Continued)

continued . . .

back soon and draws curtains around Frank's bed for privacy, leaving a space to come back in. Lawrence washes his hands with chlorhexidine 'scrub', puts on a new disposable apron, thoroughly cleans the trolley with antiseptic, checks the contents of the sealed sterile catheter packs (male) and places one on the bottom shelf of the trolley together with other items (e.g. drainage bag, spare catheter). At the bedside Lawrence follows prescribed local aseptic procedure (e.g. wearing sterile gloves) to avoid contaminating the catheter or injuring Frank during its insertion. Before reaching the bladder, the catheter gets stuck, which gentle pressure cannot overcome so Lawrence slowly withdraws it. He explains to Frank it is best not to use force to avoid injuring him, and that he could try again with a slightly larger catheter, which is more rigid and will possibly make it easier to overcome resistance. If he would rather not go through that again, an alternative type of catheter (suprapubic) could be inserted directly into the bladder by the doctors. He might find this a more comfortable option, but it does require a small surgical procedure to fit it.

Frank opts to have a suprapubic catheter inserted by the medical team and is able to empty his bladder. Although Lawrence was unsuccessful, he passes the assessment as he followed procedure, maintained aseptic 'non-touch' technique, took care not to cause injury, kept Frank fully informed, respected his freedom of choice and was able to explain his actions. Tests show Frank has aggressive, advanced (inoperable) prostate cancer that has spread to his backbone. Three weeks later Frank dies, and Lawrence helps the staff nurse perform 'last offices', cleaning and laying out his body ready for his family to see him. Lawrence feels very grateful to Frank for allowing him to try to catheterise him despite his pain, and feels it is a great shame that Frank was not able to report symptoms before as earlier intervention might have saved him.

The case study links standards of nursing education with standardised clinical decision-making and draws parallels between the roles of student/nurse and patient. As a student there is always another assessment to pass, so your career is always 'on the line' until you eventually qualify. Even when we register as nurses, every three years we have to show our knowledge and skills are up to date and we are fit to continue practising through a revalidation process, or we can be removed from the NMC register. The reason why standards are stringent is that, for patients, it is not just careers but often their lives that are 'on the line'. It is why risks have to be minimised, and standardised clinical decision-making is a way to achieve this. Although Lawrence was unsuccessful in catheterising Frank, he maintained an aseptic technique by following the correct procedure (confirmed by passing his assessment) and he could transfer these skills in caring for others. It also alerted the medical team to relieve Frank's urinary retention with a suprapubic catheter in an alternative standardised clinical procedure that successfully bypassed Frank's urethral blockage, whilst minimising risks associated with this procedure (Yates, 2016).

Table 5.1 relates standardised clinical decision-making in carrying out a practical procedure to conceptions of nursing that nurses used to describe their professional identity (Standing, 2005, 2007, 2010a). It shows that Lawrence managed to combine the discipline of being adept in specific technical skills with interpersonal qualities in caring for Frank. It is important to emphasise this point: standardised clinical decision-making can be perceived as an impersonal, task-orientated routine, but this is not a reason for ignoring the individuality and preferences of patients on the receiving end of such procedures. Some of the less enthusiastic attitudes expressed by nursing students towards standardised decision-making are possibly due to their difficulty in linking such uniform practices to individualised patient-centred care. Lawrence understood he had a duty to try to catheterise Frank safely and effectively. This required him to apply the prescribed aseptic procedure to reduce the risk of introducing infection. He knew his duty of care did not end there as he was also attentive and responsive to Frank's concerns. After looking at Table 5.1, you have an opportunity to relate these issues to your own experience in Activity 5.2.

Conceptions of nursing	Standardised clinical decision-making
Caring	Taking care to minimise Frank's discomfort.
Listening and being there	Respecting Frank's preference for 'suprapubic' catheter rather than trying a second time via the urethral route.
Practical procedures	Demonstrating aseptic technique to insert urethral urinary catheter by following the locally approved procedure.
Knowledge and understanding	Anatomy, physiology of male urinary system; pathology of urinary retention and prostate cancer, plus catheter care.
Communicating	Explaining catheterisation, checking Frank understands and consents to Lawrence carrying out the procedure.
Patience	Waiting to allow time for anaesthetic gel to take effect, not panicking or using excess force when catheter gets stuck.
Teamwork	Alerting medical team that urethral catheter will not go in bladder.
Paperwork and electronic record	Checking procedures manual and record events in care plan.
Empathising and non-judgemental	Understanding that Frank was in pain and that catheterisation can be uncomfortable, and also potentially embarrassing.
Professional	Demonstrating knowledge, skills, attitudes and clinical competence needed to pass practical assessment.

Table 5.1: Integrating standardised clinical decision-making and conceptions of nursing

Activity 5.2   *Decision-making*

Think about the various clinical procedures that you have observed or carried out with patients, and choose one example to explore in more depth. Look at how Table 5.1 related Lawrence's attempted catheterisation of Frank to the conceptions of nursing, and draw up a similar table to cross-reference your example of standardised decision-making with the conceptions of nursing. Do you find it easy or hard to mix technical and interpersonal skills

(Continued)

continued . . .

in carrying out procedures? Do you think it is necessary to combine the two contrasting skills sets? What methods do you use to check what the patient is experiencing while carrying out a procedure? Has this resulted in you making any adjustments to the procedure or not? How helpful or unhelpful do you find it to map your clinical procedure against the conceptions of nursing?

As this activity is for you to relate the above discussion to your clinical experience, no outline answer is given.

In the next section we take a look at the national picture and how governments' health policies influence standardised clinical decision-making and the structuring of healthcare services.

Health policy and standardised clinical decision-making

Each of us has standardised rights regarding our personal freedom and protection from physical or verbal harm, and standardised responsibilities in respecting the rights of others. These are our statutory rights and obligations in legislation approved by governments in Acts of Parliament. Central government also determines health policy in the UK, which gives each person a right to National Health Service (NHS) care that is free at the point of delivery (paid for indirectly via taxation). In order to ensure public money is well spent, standards are set that hospitals and community services, and health professionals, are expected to meet through sound clinical governance. As a health professional you have a right to have a high standard of education to prepare for your role, and continuing professional development opportunities to enhance your practice. In return you have a responsibility to use effective clinical decision-making skills in high quality, evidence-based, patient-centred care.

In deciding health policy, governments make use of scientific evidence to assess the nation's health with reference to morbidity (sickness) and mortality (death) rates in the population. Under *The NHS Plan* (DH, 2000) and *NHS Outcomes Framework* (DH, 2016b), government health targets were set and health outcomes identified to continually measure progress in improving the nation's health. One health target was to reduce deaths from cancer in the under 75s by 20 per cent by the year 2010. The lifetime chance of having female breast cancer and the lifetime chance of males having prostate cancer are both 1 in 8, however there has been a 17 per cent reduction in mortality in breast cancer and just a 13 per cent reduction in mortality in prostate cancer over the last decade (Cancer Research UK, 2016). The standardised screening for early detection and treatment of female breast cancer (mammography) in the UK is widespread whereas screening for prostate cancer is not, as Frank's case study illustrates. Mammography is associated with a sensitivity (ability to detect breast cancer) of up to 90 per cent, so it is considered cost-effective for national screening, and early detection leads to earlier treatment and improved survival rates. There is a prostate-specific antigen (PSA) blood test (raised levels may be linked to prostate cancer), but it is not considered sufficiently accurate or cost-effective for routine screening of males in the UK. Early detection of prostate cancer for men such as Frank relies on them alerting health professionals as soon as they have urinary problems rather than being too embarrassed to talk about it. As nurses we need to be aware of this and offer information, advice and support to encourage men to discuss such problems, particularly the over 65s, who are at higher risk of getting prostate cancer.

Sometimes standardised health screening for early detection or prevention of ill health can be perceived as counter-productive, as the next case study of a child classified as being 'overweight' helps to illustrate.

Case study: Being told you are overweight

In August 2010 a schoolgirl, aged 11, was weighed (49 kilograms/7 stone 12 pounds) and her height measured (1.524 metres/5 feet) at school as part of the National Child Measurement Programme (NCMP). After the local NHS sent a letter saying the result indicated she was overweight, she got very upset, and her mother had difficulty getting her to eat. The aim of NCMP is to promote healthy weight for healthy living and prevent obesity, which is associated with greater health risks of diabetes, cancer and heart or liver disease (DH, 2016a). Her mother was angry that a scheme designed to promote health appeared to be actually damaging her daughter's health by encouraging her to become anorexic. The story was reported in the press with pictures of the girl, who appeared to have a nice figure and did not seem overweight. It poses questions about the validity of the test and any advice given (dieting, exercise) based on the results.

The case study highlights a potential problem with standardised screening tests and how these need to be taken into account when decision-making, especially with children. As adults we are also encouraged to keep within recommended weight guidelines according to how tall we are. Measures of weight and height are used to calculate and categorise our body mass index (BMI): less than 18.5 = underweight; 18.5–25 = healthy weight; 25.1–30 = overweight; and over 30 = obese (NHS, 2010). To calculate an adult BMI score: measure weight; measure height; divide weight by height; divide again by height. If we use the case study weight and height measurements and pretend they belong to an adult we get the following BMI score:

Weight:	*49 kilograms*
Height:	*1.524 metres*
Divide weight by height:	*49 ÷ 1.524 = 32.15223*
Divide answer by height:	*32.15223 ÷ 1.524 = 21.09*
BMI score:	*21.09 (well within 18.5–25 BMI healthy weight range)*

So if the schoolgirl had been an adult with exactly the same weight and height, she would have been classified as being well within the healthy weight range. She was classified as overweight because children's BMI scores are adjusted to what is considered the norm for a child of that age; because she was large for her age she was outside the expected norm and labelled over-weight. If the child had been just one year older with the same measurements she would have been in the healthy weight range. Health promotion encouraging healthy weight and avoiding problems of obesity is a worthwhile aim. It makes sense to educate children to help prevent problems in adulthood, and the NCMP test may be accurate in the majority of cases. However, the case study shows us that individual variations from the norm do not always mean there is something wrong with the person, and that further refinement of the tests themselves may be needed to improve their accuracy. As nurses we need to be aware of the strengths and weak-nesses of standardised tests. We also need to set an example of good health, and Activity 5.3 asks you to check your own BMI.

Activity 5.3   *Evidence-based practice and research*

Do you know what your BMI score is? In this activity you are asked to apply this standardised tool to assess your weight range and appreciate what it is like for patients on the receiving end of numerous tests and investigations. You can calculate your BMI either manually (with the help of a calculator), following the steps taken on the previous page, or by logging on to **www.nhs.uk/tools/pages/BMI-healthy-weight-calculator.aspx**, which has an interactive program for you to experiment with. You still need to input your height and weight, but it does the rest, giving you a BMI score and identified weight range (healthy or otherwise). You can choose to input figures as metres and kilograms or as feet/inches and stones/pounds (a metric conversion is done to calculate the BMI score), and you can print off results as a record to compare with your future scores. When you have done this, answer the following question: What factors can you identify that affect the accuracy of the BMI score that you have calculated, and how might you optimise its accuracy?

Some possible answers can be found at the end of the chapter.

Activity 5.3 gives you a taste of what it is like to have aspects of your individuality quantified and classified according to a standardised assessment tool. As we have seen, it is important to appre-ciate the human stories behind statistics about our health status and this is supported by government policy promoting the '6Cs' of compassionate healthcare (DH, 2012a). In the next section we look at evidence-based guidelines used in standardised decision-making.

Clinical guidelines and standardised clinical decision-making

Using standardised screening techniques to assess members of the public for potential health problems needs to be combined with effective intervention tools where required. Knowing how to do this is helped by relevant evidence-based clinical guidelines. In 2014–2015 in England there were 1.1 million hospital admissions at least partly due to drinking alcohol and there were 6831 deaths directly related to alcohol consumption. In total, alcohol problems are estimated to cost the NHS a staggering £3.5 billion annually (HSCIC, 2016). The following case study describes a student who has begun to have problems with alcohol and how standardised 'AUDIT' evidence-based clinical guidelines are applied by a nurse practitioner.

Case study: Acknowledging problems with alcohol use

Anne, aged 20, is a second-year student at university studying hospitality management and hoping to work in hotels around the world. During term time Anne works part-time in the student union bar, and during the vacation she works in the cocktail bar of a restaurant. Anne enjoys drinking alcohol, her favourite being a 'Cuban' cocktail of spiced rum, cola and lime juice. Over the last year Anne has increased her alcohol consumption not just when she goes out with friends but also when she is serving drinks at the bar, and when she is alone in her room.

Anne's use of alcohol is changing from pleasant social drinking to hazardous and potentially harmful drinking. She is warned about drinking too much by the bar manager, who notices her speech is slurred; she is late for lectures and fails assignments, gets drunk at parties, strips off clothes and kisses her friend's boyfriend. Her family are very concerned about her. Then she suffers cuts and bruises when she loses control of her motorbike, and crashes into a lamp post after nightclubbing. She faces prosecution for riding a motorbike while three times over the limit of permitted alcohol. Anne is seen at the Accident and Emergency centre, and is advised to attend the university medical centre to discuss further medical care and support.

At the university medical centre, Anne is seen by Penny, a nurse practitioner, who asks what the problem is.

Anne explains about her road traffic accident, the impending prosecution and how everything generally seems to be going 'pear-shaped' in her life. Penny tells Anne she cannot change what has happened, but recognising that something is 'pear-shaped' is a good sign because it is a starting point in deciding what changes she would like to make in her life. Penny suggests it would be useful to assess Anne's alcohol consumption, which they can do together or Anne can do it independently if she prefers. Anne agrees to complete an Alcohol Use Disorders Identification Test (AUDIT) (Babor et al., 2001) with Penny. There are ten questions ranging from 'How often do you have a drink containing alcohol?' to 'Has a relative or friend or a doctor or another health worker been concerned about your drinking or suggested you cut down?' Each question has a choice of answers that are scored from 0 to 4. Scores of up to 7 out of 40 relate to lower risk sociable drinking; scores of 8–15 indicate an increased risk of drinking being hazardous to health; scores of 16–19 indicate a higher risk of drinking being harmful to oneself or others; and scores of 20 or more out of 40 indicate a higher risk of alcohol dependence that a person may need specialist help to deal with. Anne scores 26 out of 40 and is shocked to find that her average weekly consumption of 60 units of alcohol (1 litre of rum [40 units] plus two bottles of 13 per cent strength wine [20 units]) is more than four times the recommended level of 14 units of alcohol a week (ALC, 2016).

Anne questions the validity of the AUDIT assessment tool, so Penny explains it is research based and is endorsed by major healthcare organisations, including the World Health Organization (WHO), the

(Continued)

continued . . .

NHS and NICE, as an effective predictor of alcohol disorders. Anne asks what the difference is between hazardous drinking, harmful drinking and alcohol dependence. Penny replies that hazardous drinking means taking risks with personal health and safety (e.g. getting drunk), while harmful drinking means that ill health or injury occurs (e.g. motorbike crash when over alcohol limit) and alcohol dependence means knowing excessive drinking is harmful but not being able to stop doing it. Penny tells Anne that her answers indicate she should cut down her alcohol intake because drinking at her current level is associated with a higher risk of experiencing drink-related problems. She asks Anne whether her feeling that life is going 'pear-shaped' might be related to her alcohol use, and Anne agrees she tends to get into trouble when she's drunk. Penny advises Anne to aim to keep within recommended levels, for example, up to half a standard size bottle of rum (i.e. 350 ml = 14 units) or up to one and a half bottles of 12 per cent strength wine (13.5 units) a week, so she can enjoy a drink without getting so drunk she gets into trouble. Anne says she will aim to do that and put the money she saves towards repairing her motorbike so she can sell it if she gets banned and buy a push bike instead. Penny and Anne agree to meet up again in two weeks to review progress and see whether any further support or specialist referral is needed.

The standardised AUDIT assessment tool has been validated as an accurate, cost-effective way of screening and detecting alcohol problems (NICE, 2010a). It elicits information from the patient/service user for evidence of alcohol use that is then mapped against lower risk or higher risk units of alcohol consumption. This provides the basis of a 'brief intervention' where the practitioner, without judging the person, ensures they understand the health risks associated with harmful drinking (injury, high blood pressure, cancer, liver disease, relationship problems), the advisability of reducing alcohol use – enabling them to make an informed choice about the need to cut down – and the possible consequences of not doing so. In Activity 5.4 you are asked to complete an alcohol use self-assessment.

Activity 5.4   *Evidence-based practice and research*

Alcohol-related health problems are common in the UK, so it is important nurses understand initial screening tests, interventions and how units of alcohol are measured. To complete this activity, log on to **www.nhs.uk/oneyou/drinking** where you will find a box entitled 'Alcohol Checker'. Click on 'Learn more' and you will find an interactive self-assessment form entitled 'What did you drink in the last 7 days?' This is a modified 'user friendly' version of the AUDIT assessment tool that any member of the public can use. You are asked whether you drank alcohol or not on each of the last 7 days and you respond by clicking 'I didn't drink' or 'I did drink'. (If you do not drink alcohol, you could 'create' a character that does and answer questions accordingly.) Where you click 'I did drink' you will be shown a range of drinks and asked to confirm details on the type (e.g. beer, wine), size of serving, number of glasses consumed and strength of alcohol contents. When you have finished inputting information for one type of drink click 'That's it'. If you drank other types of alcohol on the same day repeat the above process. When you have entered all the

continued . . .

details for that day click 'That's it' once more and you will be directed to the next day until all seven days have been accounted for. At the end of the form you are asked for your gender and age before clicking on 'Calculate'. You will then be told how many units of alcohol your answers indicate you consumed and which category this places you in (lower risk, increased risk or higher risk). You will also be told how many calories the alcohol contained and how much money it is estimated to have cost. There are links to further information, advice and support including a 'drinks tracker app' which can be downloaded onto to a smart phone. If you want to find out more about the AUDIT questionnaire used in the case study go to **www.alcohollearningcentre.org.uk/Topics/Latest/AUDIT-Alcohol-Use-Disorders-Identification-Test** where you can open and/or download an AUDIT questionnaire (doc – 119 Kb) or the full version of AUDIT (doc – 172 Kb). Once you have finished the self-assessment, please answer the following question. What might be the limitations of the 'Alcohol Checker' self-assessment and AUDIT assessment?

Some possible answers can be found at the end of the chapter.

Activity 5.4 gave you an opportunity to test a standardised assessment tool used to diagnose whether a person's health is at risk from their pattern of alcohol consumption. In doing so you were experiencing how the health policy of reducing preventable diseases, associated with certain lifestyle choices, is linked to evidence-based tools to help people understand this and to support them in making healthier decisions. Standardised tools can also be used to prevent healthcare professionals from harming their patients by making them more aware of risks and taking steps to control them, as the following case study illustrates.

Case study: Surgeon introduces safety checklist

Atul, a well-respected surgeon in America, was operating on a patient using a procedure he had done numerous times before without incident, when he accidentally cut a main artery with the scalpel, causing a massive haemorrhage. Atul and the surgical team had only a couple of minutes to save the patient's life by finding and clamping the source of the haemorrhage, replacing lost blood and body fluids, and repairing the damaged artery. They could then go on to complete the scheduled operation. The patient survived but lost the sight of one eye, which had been deprived of oxygen as a result of the haemorrhage. This incident prompted Atul to learn from it and review ways of enhancing the prevention, control and management of potential risks in surgical procedures (Gawande, 2011).

As well as haemorrhaging, Atul was aware of many other potential risks associated with surgery, including: problems with anaesthesia; infection of wound site; operating on the wrong patient; operating on the right patient but the wrong site (e.g. removing left instead of right kidney). He looked at how other professions managed everyday uncertainties and controlled risks to human safety, while

(Continued)

continued . . .

performing highly complex activities. He discovered that pilots referred to checklists routinely during planned 'pause moments' to review specific aspects of aircraft safety before proceeding to the next critical stage (e.g. cabin doors closed before take-off). Atul noted that while each step seemed fairly straightforward, if overlooked, it could be catastrophic. He was also intrigued by research where intensive care unit nurses were asked to prompt doctors to follow a five-step checklist of questions – such as '1. Wash hands with soap' – to prevent infection by using an aseptic technique when inserting a central line (catheter in large vein near heart). Within three months, reported central line infections fell by 66 per cent, and after 18 months it was estimated that 1500 lives and $175 million had been saved (Pronovost et al., 2006). Atul began to think checklists could be effective in controlling risks in operating theatres, and he was asked by the World Health Organization (WHO) to lead an international team in promoting safe surgery globally.

Atul and his team identified three critical 'pause moments' for members of the surgical team to stop and check vital safety considerations before continuing with the next stage.

1. *Before anaesthetic is given (e.g. check identity/surgical procedure/site/consent, fit pulse oximeter to check patient's oxygen, check allergies, check if blood loss risk is >500 ml).*
2. *Before an incision is made (e.g. confirm team know each other's names/roles, action plan, availability of sterile instruments, if prophylactic antibiotics given in last 60 minutes).*
3. *Before patient leaves theatre (e.g. record procedure, nurse leads review of instruments/swab count, surgeon/anaesthetist/nurse review aloud concerns about patient recovery).*

The above became the basis of a 19-point checklist in guidelines for safe surgery (WHO, 2009). It was trialled by surgical teams in America, Canada, England, India, Jordan, New Zealand, the Philippines and Tanzania from 2007 to 2008. Death rates and complications were compared before and after introducing the checklist: before (3733 patients operated on), death rate = 1.5 per cent (56), complications = 11 per cent (410); after (3955 patients operated on), death rate = 0.8 per cent (31), complications = 7 per cent (277) (Haynes et al., 2009). So significantly fewer people died or suffered complications (e.g. infection) after the safe surgery checklist was adopted.

These death rates may seem to be relatively low, even before introducing the checklist, but it is estimated that 234 million surgical operations occur worldwide every year (Haynes et al., 2009), so a death rate of 1.5 per cent equates to 3,510,000 deaths and a death rate of 0.8 per cent equates to 1,872,000 deaths. It suggests that adopting the safe surgery checklist throughout the world could result in 1,638,000 (3,510,000 – 1,872,000) fewer surgery-related deaths each year. Because Atul had the humility to acknowledge his mistakes as a surgeon, and his dependence on the team to ensure surgery is successful (and deal with untoward incidents), he helped to create a safer system to guide surgical procedures and manage risks associated with them. In addition, he acknowledged the vital role of theatre nurses in co-ordinating the supply and monitoring of sterile instruments and equipment to minimise risks (e.g. surgeon leaving swabs inside a patient's body). Activity 5.5 asks you to think of examples of standardised procedures used to protect patients.

Activity 5.5   *Team working*

Part of the success of the safe surgery checklist in the case study is that it galvanises nurses, anaesthetists, technicians and surgeons into a team who communicate and value each other's contribution to safe and successful surgery for patients. Take a moment to think about potential risks to patients' health and safety while receiving care and treatment in clinical areas that you have worked in. What examples of standardised guidelines can you identify that are used by team members to minimise these risks and protect patients from harm? Discuss your thoughts with colleagues and your mentor.

As this is for you to review experience, no outline answer is given.

Much of the time nurses work as part of a healthcare team, and Activity 5.5 has encouraged you to think about how different team members are influenced by the same guidelines or procedures. The application of standardised health and safety guidelines is undermined if one or more team members do not adhere to them. For example, in 2010 a theatre nurse was struck off the NMC register for impairment of her fitness to practise when she was held responsible for wrongly confirming all instruments were accounted for before a patient was sewn back up. The patient had a 7-inch pair of forceps left in the abdomen and required further surgery to remove them. This example emphasises the point made earlier that our careers as nurses are always 'on the line' because patients' lives depend on us doing our jobs competently. By following standardised, evidence-based clinical decision-making we can offer higher levels of safety in controlling risks to patients' health, minimise lapses in concentration or errors of judgement (e.g. drug calculation errors) and thereby enhance our professional competence. In Chapter 6, we will look in more detail at assessing and managing risk, which includes applying 'standardised' clinical guidelines.

Chapter summary

In this chapter we looked at standardised clinical decision-making, which involves team members uniformly and consistently following agreed practical procedures, core care plans, integrated care pathways, local and national policy and evidence-based clinical guidelines. The strengths of standardised clinical decision-making include: (i) avoiding 'reinventing the wheel' by using an evidence-based protocol or checklist to guide and quality-assure assessment, planning and delivery of specific aspects of care; (ii) promoting multidisciplinary teamwork and integrated healthcare; (iii) prompting nurses and others to remember to carry out each stage of a clinical procedure in the correct sequence to avoid forgetting things and making mistakes; and (iv) recognising and controlling health risks to ensure safe and effective patient care. Weaknesses of

(Continued)

continued . . .

standardised clinical decision-making include the possibility of its uncritical application in task-orientated care that does not make patient-centred adjustments for individual differences. To optimise the strengths and minimise the limitations of standardised clinical decision-making, observation, collaborative decision-making and systematic decision-making (Chapters 2–4) need to be combined with it.

Activities: brief outline answers

Activity 5.3: Evidence-based practice and research (page 84)

You may have included the following points.

- Accuracy of equipment (scales, tape measure/height chart).
- Use of equipment, e.g. standing up straight when measured.
- Other variables, e.g. removing heavy clothing and shoes.
- Honesty of self-reporting.
- Arithmetic skills in calculating BMI.
- Variations in body types, e.g. muscular = high BMI score.

Activity 5.4: Evidence-based practice and research (pages 86–7)

You may have included the following points.

- Impaired recollection of alcohol use.
- Difficulty converting different drinks into units of alcohol.
- Ineffectiveness if person is intoxicated.
- Honesty of self-reporting.
- Possibly insufficiently motivated to change.
- Need for extra criteria to assess very high dependency.
- Alcohol Checker only covers seven days which may not accurately reflect regular drinking habit.

Further reading

Gawande, A (2011) *The checklist manifesto: how to get things right.* London: Profile Books.

An excellent read that is full of fascinating true stories, such as reviving a child who has drowned, and how standardised checklists enable us to simplify and organise complex, life-saving decisions.

Young, S and Pitcher, B (2016) *Medicines management for nurses at a glance.* Chichester: Wiley/Blackwell.

Concise, informative and well-illustrated guide to enhance understanding of medicines management in all nursing pathways and linked to NMC Standards and competencies.

Useful websites

www.gov.uk/government/organisations/department-of-health

Department of Health website where you can look at the government's health policies and planned reforms of the NHS, and access archives of previous governments' policies.

www.nhs.uk/Tools/Pages/Toolslibrary.aspx?Tag=Self+assessments&Page=1

Part of the NHS Choices website providing a wide range of evidence-based, standardised self-assessment tools/apps enabling members of the public to participate in monitoring and understanding their health needs.

www.nhs.uk/oneyou#x2sB8X7tXXQyYr8A.97

Focuses upon how lifestyle habits and choices (e.g. eating, drinking alcohol, smoking) and the ability to manage stress affects a person's health and provides support and guidance in changing lifestyle decisions.

www.nice.org.uk

National Institute for Health and Care Excellence website where you can search for quality standards and evidence-based clinical guidelines in all aspects of nursing and healthcare.

Chapter 6
Prioritising decisions in delivering care

NMC Standards for Pre-registration Nursing Education

This chapter will address the following competencies:

Domain 3: Nursing practice and decision-making
7. All nurses must be able to recognise and interpret signs of normal and deteriorating mental and physical health and respond promptly to maintain or improve the health and comfort of the service user, acting to keep them and others safe.
9. All nurses must be able to recognise when a person is at risk and in need of extra support and protection and take reasonable steps to protect them from abuse.

Domain 4: Leadership, management and team working
3. All nurses must be able to identify priorities and manage time and resources effectively to ensure the quality of care is maintained or enhanced.

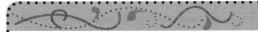

NMC Essential Skills Clusters

This chapter will address the following ESCs:

Cluster: Organisational aspects of care
9. People can trust the newly registered graduate nurse to treat them as partners and work with them to make a holistic and systematic assessment of their needs; to develop a personalised plan that is based on mutual understanding and respect for their individual situation promoting health and wellbeing, minimising risk of harm and promoting their safety at all times.

19. People can trust the newly registered graduate nurse to work to prevent and resolve conflict and maintain a safe environment.

Chapter aims

By the end of this chapter, you should be able to:

*   explain prioritising in clinical decision-making;
*   outline healthcare priorities in government policy;

- organise decision-making priorities in emergency situations;
- outline decision-making priorities in de-escalating aggression;
- explain decision-making priorities in long-term care.

Introduction

If someone asks 'What are your priorities in life?', they are trying to find out what your personal beliefs and values are regarding what you think is important, and how this influences what you choose to do. As nurses, the priorities and professional values underpinning our clinical practice are spelt out in *The Code: professional standards of practice and behaviour for nurses and midwives*, which says in the introduction:

> *The Code contains a series of statements that taken together signify what good nursing and midwifery practice looks like. It puts the interests of patients and service users first, is safe and effective, and promotes trust through professionalism.*
> (NMC, 2015, p3)

The standards we are required to meet in delivering nursing care are organised under four headings: (i) prioritise people; (ii) practise effectively; (iii) preserve safety; and (iv) promote professionalism and trust (NMC, 2015). Our main priority, therefore, is to understand the health and social care needs of people we are caring for in order to address their problems safely, effectively and professionally in partnership with them, thereby justifying the public's trust in our ability to help them. This chapter explores prioritising the health and wellbeing of patients in relation to nurses' clinical decision-making. We start by clarifying the terminology with reference to research into nursing students' perceptions of clinical decision-making skills. Relevant healthcare policy priorities are outlined, together with their implications for nursing decisions. We then discuss clinical decision-making priorities in dealing with emergency situations, in preventing and resolving conflict and aggression in clinical areas and in supporting long-term carers.

Clarifying terminology

'Prioritising' was one of ten clinical decision-making skills identified when researching students' developmental journey from the start of their programme to their first year as registered nurses (Standing, 2005, 2007, 2010a). Many of the students had worked as healthcare assistants before and recognised that some patients are less able to take care of themselves than others. They associated prioritising with assessing dependency levels and giving extra help to those who needed it most. **Prioritising in decision-making** was associated with life-saving (nurses intervening in emergency situations) as well as with recognising environmental hazards and preventing accidents from occurring.

In order to gain the public's trust in our ability to care for their health and wellbeing, we need to use prioritising skills in assessing and managing risks to their personal safety. In the following case study a nursing student describes his understanding of risk assessment.

```
. . . . . . . . . . . . . . . . . . . . . . . . . . . . . . . . . . . . . . . . . . .
```

Case study: Risk assessment and life choices

Mark is a social science graduate who volunteered on a 'nightline' service offering support to students while at university. He recently started a pre-registration nursing programme. When Mark was asked about his understanding of decision-making, and how he goes about making personal decisions, he described his view of assessing and managing potential risks.

'In risk assessment I suppose the idea is you multiply how likely something is to happen by how bad it would be. It is difficult to assign values to that kind of thing, but if you go skydiving, what are the odds of something going wrong and how bad would it be? If you go to a skydiving school, the odds are one in something very large that something would go wrong. On the other hand, if something does go wrong and you're a mile up, then it's likely to be pretty bad, so I don't think I'll be a skydiver! You can use the same process to assess other risks. My dad is having a bit of a "wonder" at the moment because he's always ridden a motorbike – and he's got a really nice one – but three things have gone wrong, and it's costing him so much to get it repaired. He feels guilty about having a motorbike and spending too much on it when he should just get a little car because it would be safer and it wouldn't cost so much. It's like risk assessment the other way round: you take how much pleasure something gives you, then minus how much it costs you.'

```
. . . . . . . . . . . . . . . . . . . . . . . . . . . . . . . . . . . . . . . . . . .
```

The case study indicates that there are potential risks associated with possible hazards in many of the life choices we make, so it makes sense to prioritise risk assessment when deciding what we are going to do. Mark's account of risk assessment and management highlights its key features:

(i) Predicting and managing uncertainty (i.e. things you cannot be totally sure about).

(ii) Recognising that some life choices carry more health risks than others (e.g. motorbike versus car).

(iii) Identifying the worst case scenario, what could go wrong (e.g. parachute fails to open).

(iv) Recognising risks to life, health and wellbeing if the worst case scenario occurs.

(v) Estimating the probability that something might go wrong (e.g. relevant injury/death rates).

(vi) Maximising safety to minimise harm when taking risks (e.g. training, checking equipment).

(vii) Weighing up costs (e.g. health risks, financial) against benefits (e.g. freedom, fun).

(viii) Being accountable for deciding whether cost outweighs benefit or benefit outweighs cost.

These principles can be applied to identify hazards and assess health risks in any setting. As nurses it is important for us to appreciate how much uncertainty is associated with what we do every day. We need to 'keep on our toes' regarding potential problems (e.g. risk of cross-infection) and avoid being complacent (e.g. forgetting to wash our hands with antiseptic scrub before and after attending to each patient). Benefits of being vigilant in this respect include: active promotion of health and prevention or lessening the effects of illness or injury; patients being confident in our ability to look after them properly; and increased confidence for us that we are doing everything we can to ensure safety of patients. Prioritising decisions in delivering nursing care, therefore, is closely linked with risk assessment and management, and for the purposes of this chapter the following definition is used.

Prioritising in decision-making applies risk assessment and management to: the immediate care of patients with life-threatening illness or injury; addressing patients' most urgent needs first; health promotion for vulnerable groups; and the avoidance of harm to patients in care settings.

In Activity 6.1 you are asked to apply prioritising and risk assessment in reflecting on and exploring a pastime, activity or event that you have participated in.

Activity 6.1   *Reflection*

This activity is intended to help you relate prioritising and risk assessment in decision-making to your own life experience. It also highlights aspects of health promotion in relation to healthy lifestyles and preventing accidents and injuries, which is relevant to nurses' preventative role. As nurses we focus on caring for patients, but if we do not look after ourselves, we will be less able to help others. Hence we need to think about how to enhance our health and wellbeing.

Think about the personal choices you make about your life, apart from choosing to study to be a nurse. These could include hobbies, keeping fit, attending social events, holidays, shopping trips, or simply your usual mode of transport in getting from one place to another. Choose one to which you can apply the above risk assessment features. Go through features (i) to (viii), relate each one to your chosen activity and write down your responses – for example, (i) anticipated uncertainty and possible risks associated with the activity and how appealing or worrying you find this. When you have finished, try to think of at least one thing you might do to enhance your own personal health and safety, and implement this in future activities if you can.

Some possible answers can be found at the end of the chapter.

So far, in clarifying the terminology we have established that prioritising in clinical decision-making is closely associated with assessing and managing health risks in individual patients, and in comparing different patients' levels of dependency We have also looked at the importance of promoting health and preventing ill health or injury to patients and the wider public both within and beyond clinical settings. These issues are also reflected in healthcare policy.

Healthcare policy priorities and implications

Promoting health and preventing ill health

Promoting health and preventing ill health are clearly desirable goals in health and social policy, as unnecessary suffering is prevented. It is also more cost-effective as less money is required for expensive hospital investigations, treatment, medicine and ongoing care. Nurses traditionally have contact with patients when illness or injury has already occurred. In this case preventative care is focused on avoiding complications to facilitate a speedy recovery (secondary prevention) or limiting the severity of long-term effects (tertiary prevention). There are now increasing opportunities for us to work in community care settings where we can be involved in *primary prevention,* for example, immunising children against mumps, measles and rubella (MMR), running clinics to help people give up smoking and providing free NHS health checks for the over 40s.

Health policy in the twenty-first century has placed increasing emphasis on health promotion and illness prevention. *The NHS Plan* (DH, 2000) outlined a strategy to reduce deaths from the main causes, such as coronary heart disease or stroke and cancer. Health targets were set to increase public access to services, reduce waiting times and offer early medical intervention. This appears to have contributed to a decline in the number of deaths despite the UK population increasing from 58.7 million in 1999 to 65.1 million in 2015. For example, the total number of deaths occurring in England and Wales was 556,118 in 1999 and by 2015 the number of deaths had fallen by nearly 5 per cent to 529,655 (ONS, 2016a). Table 6.1 summarises the main causes and numbers of deaths occurring in England and Wales in 2015.

Underlying causes of death	Number of deaths occurring
All causes (19 categories from infections to accidents)	529,655 (100% of all deaths)
Neoplasms (i.e. all cancers)	147,757 (28% of all deaths)
Diseases of the circulatory system (e.g. heart disease, stroke)	138,614 (26% of all deaths)
Diseases of the respiratory system (e.g. pneumonia)	75,534 (14% of all deaths)
Mental and behavioural disorder (e.g. dementia)	48,317 (9% of all deaths)

Table 6.1: Main underlying causes of death in England and Wales, 2015

Source: Adapted from ONS (2016a)

Table 6.1 shows that despite a reduction in the number of deaths from 1999 to 2015, over half (54 per cent) of all deaths were still due to the two main causes (cancer and circulatory disease). Hence there is scope to reduce the incidence of these and other causes of death via health promotion, education and preventative healthcare. Lord Darzi, a practising surgeon, led an NHS review that emphasised the need to *create an NHS that helps people to stay healthy* (DH, 2008a, p2) rather than treat diseases which could have been prevented by healthier lifestyle choices. Six priorities for primary care trusts (GP surgeries, health centres, practice/community nurses) to focus on were:

- tackling obesity;
- reducing alcohol harm;
- treating drug addiction;

- reducing smoking rates;
- improving sexual health;
- improving mental health.

In Activity 6.2 you are asked to think about how reducing health risks associated with these priorities might help reduce the number of deaths from the two main killers identified earlier.

Activity 6.2   *Critical thinking*

At first glance, some of the above health risks may not seem obviously linked to the two main killer diseases. However, take time to look at each priority in turn, and think about how achieving these might also help to reduce deaths from cancer or circulatory diseases. Try to identify possible physiological changes associated with each health risk listed and link these to effects on the heart, circulation or cancer sites. You might then get an idea of how tackling these priorities can help to reduce the two main causes of death.

Some possible answers can be found at the end of the chapter.

Activity 6.2 highlights areas of health promotion and illness prevention that nurses can engage in regarding informing, advising and supporting people to get fit and stay healthy. Out-patient, community and practice nurses also help people manage various conditions (e.g. diabetes, asthma, high blood pressure, mental health issues) to prevent relapses and reduce hospital readmissions.

Providing high quality care

While promoting health and preventing ill health have, in recent years, been recognised as key priorities, much of our work as nurses will also be focused on caring for acutely ill patients or those with long-term medical conditions. Government policy in relation to healthcare, in hospital or community settings, prioritises patients' rights to receive a high quality service. Standardised clinical guidelines, as discussed in Chapter 5, are designed to enable a high standard of care to be consistently delivered.

> *High quality care should be as safe and effective as possible, with patients treated with compassion, dignity and respect. As well as clinical quality and safety, quality means care that is personal to each individual.*
> (DH, 2008a, p7)

You might be surprised that such fairly straightforward principles should require a high level government-led review. After all, is it not simply saying we should treat people as human beings, care for them, protect them from harm and help them get better? It is not exactly a 'cutting edge' revelation, is it? The problem is that there have, in recent years, been several well-publicised examples of appalling standards of unsafe, ineffective, uncaring and dehumanising healthcare in the NHS and private sectors. Such cases can undermine all the good work that is done and the public's confidence in the NHS as a whole. Part of the explanation why some hospitals veered away from such basic healthcare values was that they were preoccupied with meeting health targets such as getting more patients assessed and treated more quickly, but they failed to adequately manage the resource implications. This led to overstretched services with staff not coping with demands, and patient care being neglected.

When problems occur in the organisation and delivery of healthcare, the priority is to learn from it and make changes to prevent such things from happening again. In effect, the above definition of high quality care summarises values found in nurses' and other health professionals' ethical codes of practice. Lord Darzi's NHS review team argued that these values need to be applied by everyone working in health and social care, including NHS Trust executives and managers who are responsible for monitoring the quality of care. All healthcare personnel are required to pledge their ongoing commitment to these values, which are enshrined in a new NHS Constitution (see Chapter 10). This represents a contract between healthcare providers and the public, and future funding is dependent on fulfilling the agreed terms in delivering high quality care.

Government health policy priorities in recent years have increasingly focused on (i) health promotion to prevent ill health associated with obesity, smoking, alcohol and drug misuse; (ii) providing higher standards of safe, effective and compassionate care; and (iii) being more patient-centred and publicly accountable for the quality of care that we provide. In order to evaluate healthcare organisations' and professionals' achievements, an *NHS Outcomes Framework* was proposed to identify measurable performance indicators, for example, patient-reported outcome measures (PROMs), regarding five key domains (priorities):

Domain 1: Preventing people from dying prematurely.

Domain 2: Enhancing quality of life for people with long-term conditions.

Domain 3: Helping people recover from episodes of ill health or following injury.

Domain 4: Ensuring people have a positive experience of care.

Domain 5: Treating and caring for people in a safe environment and protecting them from avoidable harm.

(DH, 2016b)

As nurses we have a duty to help to achieve each of these priorities. Activity 6.3 asks you to think about what we might contribute, and how our interventions might be evaluated.

Activity 6.3   *Reflection and decision-making*

Look at the five domains of the *NHS Outcomes Framework*. For each one, try to identify at least one example of what nurses can do to achieve it and how to measure outcomes of care.

Some possible answers can be found at the end of the chapter.

Activity 6.3 links the clinical challenges that nurses and other health professionals have to deal with every day (through promoting health, preventing ill health and endeavouring to deliver high quality care) to government health policy priorities. The main difference between these priorities which focus upon patient outcomes and previous health targets is that there is greater emphasis on:

- patients' experience and outcomes of care, rather than assuming increasing numbers of people accessing the NHS results in quality care;
- identifying more meaningful patient-centred indicators, such as PROMs, to audit the quality of care;
- assessing, managing and controlling risks to patients' safety in the clinical environment itself, such as preventing cross-infection and injuries;
- integrating health and social care in the community to support those with long-term conditions or disabilities to enable them to enjoy a good quality of life.

The priorities in the five domains of the *NHS Outcomes Framework* also place more emphasis on NHS Trust executives and managers enabling health professionals to give high quality patient-centred care by ensuring adequate staffing levels, training and equipment. In turn, health professionals are expected to consult and collaborate with patients (see Chapter 2), as there should be *no decision about me, without me* (DH, 2012b). The development and application of PROMs also take patient empowerment a step further than before because the performance of nurses and other health professionals is, in effect, evaluated by the patients we care for. It underlines the importance of dealing quickly with perceived problems in the organisation or delivery of care so that any harm to patients is prevented, and any inconvenience to them is kept to a minimum.

This is consistent with the requirements of nurses' own professional *Code* regarding risk assessment and management in protecting the health and safety of patients.

Preserve safety

16 Act without delay if you believe that there is a risk to patient safety or public protection

17 Raise concerns immediately if you believe a person is vulnerable or at risk and needs extra support and protection

19 Be aware of, and reduce as far as possible, any potential for harm associated with your practice
(NMC, 2015, pp11–14)

The following scenario gives an example of how to manage risk in clinical practice.

Scenario

Imagine you are on placement in a hospital ward and you are asked to help a more senior student make a bed while the patient has gone to the bathroom. The other student uses the foot pump to elevate the bed so that neither of you has to bend down too far, making the job a bit easier. When the bed is made the senior student thanks you and says she is going for her break, but she does not let the bed down for the patient to get back in. What would you do about it?

(Continued)

continued . . .

1. *Nothing because the other student is senior to you.*
2. *Remind the other student to lower the bed there and then.*
3. *Remind the other student to lower the bed after her break.*
4. *Check again later to see whether the bed was lowered.*
5. *Lower the bed to a safe height yourself without delay.*

Try to decide what you would do in this situation before continuing this chapter.

At first glance this scenario may not seem to be a very serious health risk, but there have been a number of serious injuries and fatalities resulting from patients falling out of bed. Hospital beds are often higher up than beds at home, and floors are usually hard, not carpeted. Additional risk factors are that patients in hospital may be weaker than normal, and they could be taking medication that makes them drowsy or susceptible to injury. Ensuring that beds are a safe height for patients to get in and out of is, therefore, a health and safety priority.

In the scenario, the patient could come back from the bathroom at any time and try to get back into bed, so if it has not been lowered, the patient will have difficulties, and there is a risk they may fall down. Of the possible responses listed above, 2 and 5 are the only safe options (with 2 being preferable, as the other student might do the same thing again if her memory lapse is not brought to her attention). It is not about 'scoring points' off each other; it is about nurses being committed to ensuring that patients are safe and realising we can all make mistakes, so we need to help each other put these right. The senior student would feel guilty if the patient suffered an injury because she had forgotten to lower the bed. As nurses and health professionals we have a duty of care, which means that we all share a responsibility for maintaining a safe environment to protect patients (and ourselves) from injury. This is endorsed by health policy in creating a compassionate NHS culture by promoting the '6Cs' of care, compassion, competence, communication, courage and commitment (DH, 2012a).

The Health and Safety Executive (HSE) identifies five steps to risk assessment in the workplace (HSE, 2011), which we can relate to the above scenario as follows.

1. *Identify hazards (things that may cause harm)* – patient's bed left too high up.
2. *Decide who might be harmed and how* – patient could fall getting into bed.
3. *Evaluate risks (likelihood of injury) and decide on precautions* – increased risk of falling/being injured (e.g. fracture) so the hazard should be made safe.
4. *Record your findings and implement them* – remind colleague to lower the bed.
5. *Review your assessment and update if necessary* – check if bed-making procedure mentions leaving the bed at a safe height; if not, recommend that it does.

There are occasions when reminding colleagues of their responsibilities in protecting patients from harm does not work and they continue to put patients at risk, as in the next case study.

Case study: 'Whistleblowing'

Between November 2009 and January 2010 the NMC Conduct and Competence Committee reviewed evidence in cases raising concerns about registered nurses' fitness to practise. In one such case, two healthcare assistants gave evidence about the conduct of a registered nurse they worked with at night in a nursing home. They reported that the registered nurse routinely did not follow approved procedures in caring for the residents, which put them at risk. This included: putting double thickness incontinence pads on residents, meaning they could be left soiled for longer; failing to turn residents every two hours to prevent pressure sores despite recording in the nursing notes that they had been turned; and making a habit of sleeping while on duty. The healthcare assistants reported their concerns to the home manager, who investigated and then reported the nurse to the NMC. The NMC judged that the nurse's fitness to practise was impaired, and she was struck off the NMC register.

The case study is an example of 'whistleblowing' (in which loyalty to colleagues is secondary to protecting the health and safety of those in our care) when allegations of inappropriate, unprofessional conduct are reported verbally and in writing to the relevant authorities (e.g. managers, the NMC).

There are also times when nurses and other health professionals 'have their hands tied' in trying to manage risks where there are not sufficient resources to cope with clinical demands. This is where managers and NHS Trust executives bear some responsibility for potentially unsafe working conditions in clinical areas. Organisations such as the Health and Safety Executive (HSE) and Care Quality Commission (CQC) have statutory powers to investigate complaints about unsafe and poor quality provision in hospitals or other health and social care settings. In the earlier scenario we looked at risk management with hospital beds. In a related, real-life case, the HSE prosecuted an NHS Trust because in November 2007 an 89-year-old male patient fell out of bed and died. The HSE argued that the NHS Trust should have ensured bed safety rails were available and fitted to the sides of the patient's bed to prevent him falling, and that by failing to do so they contributed to his death. As nurses we also have a responsibility to inform managers where additional equipment is needed or current equipment needs maintaining or repairing (e.g. suction machine not working). In the next case study the CQC investigate an NHS Trust's management of a mental health unit.

Case study: Investigation into quality of care

Between October 2007 and November 2008 six patients died on a ten-bed mental health unit in a community hospital, and this prompted an investigation into the quality of care provided. The findings revealed that there was poor leadership, poor clinical governance and deficiencies in the way the unit was managed. This included inadequate supervision of doctors. For example, some doctors were prescribing

(Continued)

continued . . .

controlled drugs such as morphine or diamorphine (very powerful painkillers often used in end-of-life care to relieve suffering) inappropriately to subdue elderly, confused patients suffering from dementia. There were not enough nurses to run the unit safely, and little or no provision for staff training. There was little evidence of effective multidisciplinary teamwork or decision-making. Record keeping and care planning were also poor.

Following discussions with the CQC, the NHS Trust closed the unit in July 2009, as 'it could not guarantee sufficient staffing levels to provide a safe service.' Unfortunately this is not an isolated occurrence consigned to the historic past. A BBC Panorama *documentary film 'Nursing homes undercover' (21 November 2016) showed an elderly patient with severe dementia (in a private nursing home which charged the local authority £3000 per week for her care) being badly treated and given morphine by the nurse to 'shut her up' (see* **www.bbc.co.uk/iplayer/episode/b0844wq3/panorama-nursing-homes-undercover**). *This shows we cannot afford to become complacent.*

In Activity 6.4 you are asked to adopt the role of an investigator in relation to the case study.

Activity 6.4   *Leadership and management*

Imagine you are a member of the CQC investigation team reviewing the quality of care in the mental health unit referred to above. Look at the definition of high quality care (DH, 2008a) on page 97, and apply it in critiquing the quality of care described in the case study.

Some possible answers can be found at the end of the chapter.

In Activity 6.4 you were asked to switch perspectives from an 'insider' learning how to be a nurse to an 'outsider' looking in and critically reviewing health professionals' quality of care. In a sense, this is something we need to do continually if we are going to successfully prioritise high quality care for our patients at all times, and it will be further discussed in Chapter 10, which explores **accountability in clinical decision-making**.

This section has explored the influence of health policy in prioritising health promotion, ill health prevention and the provision of high quality patient-centred care. In the next section we look at how nurses use prioritising decision-making skills in dealing with emergency situations.

Dealing with emergency situations

Effective prioritising in clinical decision-making can mean a patient survives rather than dies from an acute life-threatening episode. As we discussed earlier, preventing people from dying prematurely is a key priority in healthcare, and circulatory disease is a major cause of death, accounting for over a quarter of deaths in England and Wales in 2015. As nurses, we need to be able to recognise when a patient needs urgent clinical intervention and know what to do about it. In the following case study a student nurse senses something is seriously wrong with a patient.

Case study: Recognising and reporting a medical emergency

Dennis is at the end of his first year as a student nurse, and he is on a practice placement in a medical ward. One of the patients he has been looking after is Roy, aged 42, who runs a taxi business and was admitted because of a recent history of severe chest pain. Roy has been advised to stop smoking. He has cut down from 20 to 10 a day but finds it too difficult to stop and he regularly goes out for a smoke while on the ward.

One day Dennis notices Roy returning from his 'outing' very slowly, looking breathless and pale, clutching his chest and grimacing. Dennis helps him onto the bed and notices he is sweating profusely. He asks Roy if he is in pain but gets no answer. Dennis tries to feel Roy's radial (wrist) pulse but cannot find it. He informs the ward manager; she takes one look at Roy and tells Dennis to dial the 'crash call' number to alert the duty resuscitation team, and then bring the resuscitation trolley to Roy's bed.

When Dennis arrives with the trolley, Roy appears unconscious and the sister is performing cardio-pulmonary resuscitation (CPR). She checks that Dennis called the 'crash' team and tells him to elevate the foot of the bed to help blood return to Roy's heart. The 'crash' team arrives (anaesthetist and physician); they help continue CPR, monitor and defibrillate (electrically stimulate) Roy's heart. He is revived, given morphine and transferred to coronary care. The sister tells Dennis he did a good job in recognising something was wrong, alerting her, alerting the 'crash' team, remaining calm and helping her by doing what she asked without hesitation. By doing so, Dennis fulfilled the professional requirements of The Code *regarding item 15 'Always offer help if an emergency arises ...' (NMC, 2015, p12).*

The case study shows that even a first-year student nurse can help prevent the premature death of a patient by: using observation skills (Chapter 3); reporting concerns and collaborating with other team members (Chapter 2); systematically identifying the problem – the absence of a radial pulse (Chapter 4); and following agreed standardised procedures for emergencies (Chapter 5) with guidance from the sister in prioritising Roy's life-threatening episode above all else. The severe pain Roy experienced is associated with myocardial infarction (MI), the death of heart muscle from oxygen deprivation caused by a blood clot or narrowing of the coronary arteries. There is a high mortality (death) rate, as 30 per cent of people experiencing MI for the first time die from it (NICE, 2010b). Survival is improved by immediate diagnosis and intervention, so nurses must recognise a heart attack and administer CPR if there is no carotid (neck) pulse or respiration, which is why the sister began CPR in the case study. In Roy's case, he also needs help to give up smoking as this puts him at risk of further heart attacks by causing blood vessels to constrict. Activity 6.5 invites you to find out more about CPR and the emergency equipment needed.

| **Activity 6.5** | *Evidence-based practice and research* |

St John Ambulance advises that all members of the public should learn how to: recognise when someone is having a heart attack; dial 999 (UK) or 112 (Europe and UK) for an ambulance; and do CPR if the patient loses consciousness, stops breathing and has no pulse. As nurses we should make it a priority to be competent in using these skills, and in checking the contents of the resuscitation trolley. Look this up by searching the literature and checking the up-to-date guidelines provided by the Resuscitation Council (UK) on their website. Practise CPR using a SimMan or manikin in a skills lab, and ask your mentor to quiz you about the resuscitation trolley contents.

As this is for you to find out about and practise, no outline answer is provided.

Activity 6.5 encourages you to develop confidence in being calm and effective when someone needs CPR, a physiological life-saving intervention. In the next section we look at prioritising in the context of psychological interventions to prevent and calm down aggressive behaviour.

Preventing and de-escalating conflict and aggression

Sometimes prioritising the protection of a patient from harm in clinical settings can involve preventing or de-escalating aggression in them, other patients, visitors or members of staff. Various factors can contribute to patients feeling angry such as: fear about what is wrong with them; previous negative experience; pain; frustration at being kept waiting; not feeling in control of what is going on; separation from friends/family; and feeling misunderstood or uncared for. Anger may escalate as aggressive shouting, verbal abuse, threats or physical abuse towards objects (e.g. slamming doors) or self (e.g. head banging) or other people (e.g. punching). In the following case study a student nurse realises he has provoked a patient to be aggressive.

Case study: Saying sorry to a patient

When Lawrence was a first-year student nurse (mental health) he was working in a rehabilitation unit. One of the patients, Cecil, aged 57, had a history of a stroke (blood clot in the brain), which resulted in him suffering muscle weakness in his left arm and leg, speech difficulties and a personality change associated with becoming aggressive and violent to others. One day Lawrence was asked by the charge nurse to call the patients to have lunch. Due to Cecil's mobility problems he was slower than the others to respond, and unthinkingly Lawrence said, 'Hurry up, Cecil, it will be cold by the time you get there!' Despite Cecil's disability he lunged at Lawrence, putting his right hand round his throat and squeezing as hard as he could. Lawrence realised he had been insensitive and impatient, looked at Cecil and said, 'I'm sorry, I was out of order.' Cecil released his grip and Lawrence walked with him (at his pace) to the dining room.

The case study shows how Lawrence's initial intervention escalated Cecil's violent behaviour and how his subsequent intervention (saying sorry) de-escalated Cecil's anger and aggression. It also helps to illustrate de-escalation interventions described by Olver (2007).

- *Active listening*: The more we are able to convey that we are interested, attentive and listening to the person's concerns, the better the chances of them ventilating feelings without becoming violent. (Part of Cecil's frustration was due to his speech impairment so there was a greater risk of him expressing anger physically rather than verbally.)
- *Acknowledging concerns*: It helps to confirm that we have understood what the person has said and why they may be feeling frustrated or angry. (Lawrence was suddenly aware that he had been insensitive and impatient and that this had, understandably, angered Cecil.)
- *Agreeing with truths*: When people are angry they are less able to reason and can get more aggressive if we try to argue a point with them. We may want to challenge any unfair comments or abusive language, but the best way we can do this is by not 'rising to the bait', otherwise we are likely to get angry too. Instead, we should try to focus on those parts of a person's tirade that may have a basis in reality regarding perceived injustice. (Lawrence did not try to argue that Cecil's reaction was too aggressive, and he did not retaliate with physical force. Instead, he understood he should have been more patient.)
- *Apologising for situation*: Where we recognise that a person has a legitimate grievance, if we convey we are sorry for what they have had to endure (without taking blame for others), their current level of aggression is more likely to subside. (In the case study, Lawrence *was* at fault, so he apologised for his behaviour, and it worked: Cecil calmed down.)
- *Inviting criticism*: Showing that we are prepared to listen to any suggestions to improve services may also reduce a person's possible sense of powerlessness and frustration. As mentioned earlier, enhancing patients' experience and both valuing and responding to their feedback are now priorities in giving quality care (DH, 2016b). (Cecil was not able to articulate his criticism, but Lawrence understood his non-verbal criticism very clearly.)

De-escalation techniques are important communication and interpersonal skills used to avoid 'adding fuel to the fire' when people are upset and angry, and all nurses need to develop and practise them. In using them, nurses need to protect themselves by ensuring that other staff are available for support and that they have an escape route should the person become more violent. At this point more specialist mental health and/or learning disability nursing skills in managing disturbed or challenging behaviour would be required (NICE, 2015a, 2015b), or the police may need to be called to physically restrain the person.

Supporting long-term carers

Prioritising decision-making in dealing with emergencies or de-escalating aggression is focused on short-term acute episodes in clinical areas that have resources intended to tackle them. As referred to earlier, the quality of long-term care is now also recognised as a priority (DH, 2016b), but this is often provided by a spouse or family member who copes alone, unaware of the support in the community that can help to improve their quality of life and ease the burden of care. In the following case study Pippa, a community nurse specialising in caring for patients with dementia, is asked by the GP to assess a couple as the husband is finding it hard to cope with his wife.

Case study: Supporting a long-term carer

Pippa visits Stan, aged 65, and Audrey, aged 60 (diagnosed with Alzheimer's disease, an early form of dementia) at their home. She introduces herself but two minutes later Audrey has forgotten who she is. Stan makes everyone a cup of tea and guides Audrey to her favourite chair to sit and listen to music while having her tea. Pippa can see Stan is caring and attentive to Audrey and asks him how long she has needed looking after in this way. Stan explains that Audrey has been like this for five years. She is very forgetful. It is upsetting if they've just got back from somewhere nice and she cannot remember anything about it. She cannot be left alone, as she wanders off and gets lost because she does not know where she is. He gave up work five years ago to take care of her, and has not had a break in that time. He looks after her 24 hours a day, seven days a week. They have two grown-up daughters who have their own families and do not live nearby; when they visit, Audrey does not recognise them. Stan says that they had had such great plans for a happy and active retirement travelling the world together, but 'that has all gone out the window now'. Their savings and pension have been depleted through Stan having to give up work early. Recently he has been feeling guilty for getting angry and shouting at her when she keeps asking the same question over and over again. Stan says he cannot go on like this for much longer, but he does not want Audrey to go into a nursing home.

Pippa discovers Stan has not claimed any disability living allowance for Audrey, and helps him do so, which relieves some of the financial worries. She identifies a mental health day centre that caters for patients such as Audrey, and she now attends three days a week. Pippa also arranges for Audrey to be admitted as an in-patient in a specialist unit for two weeks every year to give Stan a period of respite when he can explore some of the places he wants to visit. Pippa also continues to visit Stan and Audrey. Stan feels his life has been transformed: he does not feel so alone with the responsibility any more. Audrey seems happy at the mental health centre and the unit; Stan can go for walks without worrying about her; and he finds Pippa very understanding.

Carers like Stan do a tremendous job in looking after loved ones, often without having someone to share the burden with, off-duty time or even an annual holiday. They enable long-term patients to be cared for at home where possible, and reduce their dependence on expensive in-patient or residential health and social care. Supporting carers in the community is vital to enhance the patient's and carer's experience of care and their quality of life together, as demonstrated by Pippa in the case study. An emphasis on patients' experience of care in the *NHS Outcomes Framework* (DH, 2016b) also supports the application of nurses' caring qualities and skills. Table 6.2 cross-references prioritising in decision-making with nurses' conceptions of nursing in relation to the case study.

Table 6.2 also conveys how Pippa's support of Stan in caring for Audrey contributed to a 'culture of compassionate care' as advocated in government health policy (DH, 2012a), which identifies

Conceptions of nursing	Prioritising in clinical decision-making
Caring	Focusing caring on Stan in recognition of his devotion to his wife and his need for support to help him care for her.
Listening and being there	Enabling Stan to talk about the problems he faces every day to keep Audrey as safe and well cared for as he can.
Practical procedures	Implementing changes to improve Stan's quality of life, enabling him to have some time to relax and unwind.
Knowledge and understanding	Understanding changes to brain in Alzheimer's disease and their effect on cognition, memory, behaviour, mood and personality.
Communicating	Questioning Stan to assess how he is coping with Audrey, informing him of the range of services that may be of help.
Patience	Happy to keep reminding Audrey when she forgets her name.
Teamwork	Liaising with GP, mental health day centre and in-patient unit to provide alternative care for Audrey and respite for Stan.
Paperwork and electronic record	Helping Stan complete disability living allowance forms.
Empathising and non-judgemental	Stan's sense of loss at losing the wife he knew yet seeing her every day, and understanding his frustration.
Professional	Enhancing quality in safety and effectiveness of Audrey's care, her patient experience and Stan's carer experience.

Table 6.2: Integrating prioritising in clinical decision-making and conceptions of nursing

six core values/behaviour needed to provide high quality, compassionate care. These are known as the '6Cs': care, compassion, competence, communication, courage and commitment. The courage and commitment were provided by Stan, but he was enabled to continue caring for Audrey because of Pippa's 'compassionate competence' in communicating/supporting him.

Addressing patients' long-term care needs is a growing challenge as the number of people requiring support is increasing as the UK population expands. This may in part be due to improvements in health which enable people to live longer. However, this results in a larger proportion of older people who are more susceptible to age-related health and social care problems. In 2004 64.5 per cent of the population was aged 16–64 and 15.9 per cent was 65 and over. In 2024 it is estimated that 61.1 per cent of the population will be 16–64 and 19.9 per cent will be 65 and over, and this trend is set to continue (ONS, 2016b). A decline in those of working age and increase in those who have retired from work poses questions about the sustainability of an NHS funded by taxation. In order to cope with challenges associated with changing demographics and preventable ill health (obesity, smoking etc.) a reappraisal of health priorities was needed. This is reflected in the Health and Social Care Act 2012 and the *NHS Five Year Forward View* (NHS England, 2014). These emphasise the importance of prevention to limit avoidable demands for treatment; improved integration, efficiency and quality in organising and delivering health and social care; and optimising the use of precious resources (financial, personnel, buildings and equipment) to address demands. Primary, out of hospital, community-based services are therefore becoming more influential than secondary, hospital-based services in determining health and social care priorities. This is evidenced by: (i) GP-led clinical commissioning groups being responsible for identifying and purchasing healthcare for patients in their communities; (ii) local authorities being responsible for assessing and addressing social care and public health needs; (iii) greater collaboration and integration between health and social care agencies; (iv) the development of new models of care incorporating service user involvement and technological aids to enhance self-care, such as interactive programmes (see Chapter 5); and (v) local healthwatch organisations representing service users' interests.

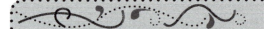

Chapter summary

This chapter explored what is meant when we talk about prioritising in clinical decision-making. Prioritising was closely linked with risk assessment and risk management, and a five-step model was described and applied (HSE, 2011). Priorities in health policy were then looked at, focusing on health promotion, ill health prevention and giving high quality patient-centred care. Mortality rates were related to policy priorities in reducing the number of premature deaths from the main killer diseases such as cancer. High quality care was defined with reference to the findings of Lord Darzi's NHS review, the *NHS Outcomes Framework* and the '6Cs' of care, compassion, competence, communication, courage and commitment (DH, 2012a). The need to adapt care priorities and strategies in light of demographic changes and rise in behaviours associated with preventable ill health was noted. The strengths of prioritising in decision-making are in focusing the attention of NHS services and health professionals to achieve desired outcomes by managing available resources effectively. The weaknesses of prioritising in decision-making are that it can distract NHS services and health professionals from attending to patients' other needs and concerns that may be just as important to them. Case studies of nurses applying prioritising in decision-making to emergency care, de-escalating aggression and supporting carers of those with long-term conditions were used to link the theory of prioritising decisions to nursing practice.

Activities: brief outline answers

Activity 6.1: Reflection (page 95)
Applying risk assessment criteria to, for example, going swimming in a public pool.

(i)   Predicting/managing uncertainty: will it be crowded? Time visit to avoid school groups.
(ii) Comparative health risks: good supervision, clearer water, less risky than sea, river or lake.
(iii) Worst case scenario: bang head or get stuck under water and lose consciousness.
(iv) Risks to life/health if (iii) occurs: death from drowning if not rescued by lifeguard.
(v)   Probability (iii) might happen: extremely unlikely, but fatalities have occurred before.
(vi) Maximising safe risk taking: don't dive in shallow end/near water outlet/if pool not clear.

(vii)   Costs versus benefits of choice: chlorine smell and sore eyes versus very good exercise.

(viii) Accountability for decision-making: don't swim if unwell; don't endanger self or others.

Activity 6.2: Critical thinking (page 97)

You may have included the following points:

1.   Tackling obesity: losing weight reduces strain on heart, cholesterol, fatty deposits in arteries (fewer heart attacks); healthy diet with five portions of fruit/vegetables daily reduces bowel cancer risk.
2.   Reducing alcohol harm: cutting down alcohol to safe limits reduces risk of cancer in throat, liver, bowel and breast; also reduces risk of obesity, high blood pressure, stroke.
3.   Treating drug addiction: reduces risk of heart failure or cocaine-induced heart attack.
4.   Reducing smoking rates: reduces risk of cancer of lung, throat and pancreas; also reduces risk of heart attacks, high blood pressure and stroke.
5.   Improving sexual health: safe sex reduces risk of cervical cancer caused by sexually transmitted human papillomavirus; report early symptoms of breast and prostate cancer.
6.   Improving mental health: reducing stress reduces levels of hormones (e.g. cortisone), which in turn reduces risk of high blood pressure, stroke or heart attack.

Activity 6.3: Reflection and decision-making (page 98)

Examples of nurses applying *NHS Outcomes Framework* domains/priorities.

Domain 1   *Preventing people from dying prematurely*: Ask doctor to prescribe anticoagulant to reduce deep vein thrombosis/pulmonary embolism risk; compare death rates before and after.

Domain 2   *Enhancing quality of life for people with long-term conditions*: Support patients and carers, co-ordinate community resources, arrange respite care; patients/carers feel supported.

Domain 3   *Helping people recover from episodes of ill health or following injury*: Help patients address activities of living to aid recuperation; competent interventions; record readmissions.

Domain 4   *Ensuring people have a positive experience of care*: Keep patients fully informed about available choices and progress, and share decision-making with them; PROMs data.

Domain 5   *Treating and caring for people in a safe environment and protecting them from avoidable harm*: Use of antiseptic hand scrub between patient contacts to minimise clinical infection rates.

Activity 6.4: Leadership and management (page 102)

You may have included the following points in your critique of care.

*   *Safety of care*: Unsafe as an unusually high proportion of the patients died; inadequate staffing levels, teamwork, supervision or management, which put patients' health and wellbeing at risk.

*   *Effectiveness of care*: Inappropriate prescribing of powerful controlled drugs militated against accurate assessment or therapeutic interventions with elderly patients who were just subdued.

*   *Compassion, dignity and respect*: Absent due to poor standards of care. Nurses (who could have advocated on patients' behalf) colluded with the treatment regime instead of challenging it.

Further reading

Fisher, M and Scott, M (2013) *Patient safety and managing risk in nursing*. London: Sage/Learning Matters.

Useful guide in creating a safe environment for patients to manage risks to their health and wellbeing by adopting procedures to minimise human error and deal with incidents effectively.

Northway, R and Jenkins, R (2017) *Safeguarding adults in nursing practice* (2nd edn). London: Sage/Learning Matters.

Applies risk assessment and management to safeguard and prioritise care for vulnerable adults, including people with learning disabilities.

Useful websites

www.cqc.org.uk

Care Quality Commission website with links to current and past investigations.

www.england.nhs.uk/nursingvision

NHS website prioritising compassion in practice within a culture of compassionate care. It contains useful resources and downloads regarding the '6Cs' and how they can be applied in different pathways.

www.hse.gov.uk

Health and Safety Executive website describing its role and function.

www.resus.org.uk

The Resuscitation Council (UK) website has up-to-date guidelines on resuscitation.

www.sja.org.uk

St John Ambulance website, full of useful first aid information.

Chapter 7
Experience and intuition in decision-making

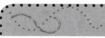

NMC Standards for Pre-registration Nursing Education

This chapter will address the following competencies:

Domain 3: Nursing practice and decision-making

5. All nurses must understand public health principles, priorities and practice in order to recognise and respond to the major causes and social determinants of health, illness and health inequalities. They must use a range of information and data to assess the needs of people, groups, communities and populations, and work to improve health, wellbeing and experiences of healthcare; secure equal access to health screening, health promotion and healthcare; and promote social inclusion.

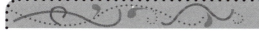

NMC Essential Skills Clusters

This chapter will address the following ESCs:

Cluster: Care, compassion and communication

1. As partners in the care process, people can trust a newly registered graduate nurse to provide collaborative care based on the highest standards, knowledge and competence.

10. People can trust the newly registered graduate nurse to deliver nursing interventions and evaluate their effectiveness against the agreed assessment and care plan.

18. People can trust a newly registered nurse to enhance the safety of service users and identify and actively manage risk and uncertainty in relation to people, the environment, self and others.

Chapter aims

By the end of this chapter, you should be able to:

- describe how experience and intuition influence decision-making;
- explain the meaning of tacit (embodied/embedded) knowledge and skills;
- relate experience and intuition to examples of clinical decision-making;
- discuss the pros and cons of experience and intuition in decision-making.

Introduction

Of all the clinical decision-making skills discussed in this book, experience and intuition are the most vague and difficult to describe. Common sense suggests they are an important influence as we tend to be much more effective two months into a practice placement than on our first day. We also come across experienced nurse role models who somehow seem to know how to deal with challenging situations.

We are continually adding to our experience as nurses while trying to ensure that patients have a *good experience* of healthcare – this being a health policy priority (Chapter 6) that is reflected in the NMC *Standards for pre-registration nursing education* (2010). To give person-centred care we need to understand and respond to each patient as an individual who experiences things in their own unique way. In order to do this we need to draw on our personal and professional experience and intuition to empathise and communicate with patients, and adapt decision-making and nursing procedures to their particular circumstances.

The following case study links a positive childhood patient experience with becoming a nurse.

Case study: Childhood memory of being nursed

Soon after Simon started a pre-registration nursing programme he was asked about his reasons for becoming a nurse. In response, he described an incident he experienced as a young child.

'When I was three I was chasing after my brother in the garden when I tripped outside the greenhouse, breaking a pane of glass as I fell, and my arm was bleeding a lot. My mum rushed me to casualty where I had to have an injection and stitches as the wound in my arm was cleaned, sewn up and bandaged. The nursing staff were so pleasant and polite, especially a male nurse who bandaged up my teddy bear.'

The case study suggests that the nurses made a special effort to ensure young Simon had a positive experience of emergency care while also attending to his wound competently. Twenty-two years later the incident was still vivid in Simon's memory, and the nurse he encountered as a child represents an early role model that he now aspires to emulate. Activity 7.1 asks you to reflect on this nurse's decision-making as described in the case study.

Activity 7.1   *Reflection*

Read through the introduction to this chapter and the case study again, and then write down your answers to the following questions.

1. What was the point of the male nurse bandaging young Simon's teddy bear?
2. What impact did this nurse's intervention appear to have on Simon?
3. What can be learnt from this incident that might also apply to adult care?

Some possible answers can be found at the end of the chapter.

The case study reinforces the idea that previous experience influences subsequent decisions, as Simon's childhood experience contributed to his decision to study nursing years later. We do not know how the male nurse developed his understanding of children. It could relate to his own childhood memories, his experience of parenthood or working with children or the study of developmental psychology. Whatever influenced him, it led to a spontaneous, intuitive decision to bandage the teddy bear in addition to the standardised wound dressing procedure. This appeared useful in complementing the physical aspects of care with psychological support. We often tap into previous life experience to guide our intuitive judgement and decision-making, but we also need to recognise when we are 'out of our depth' and lack the necessary experience to deliver nursing care competently (see the Essential Skills Clusters at the start of this chapter).

This chapter explains what experience and intuition in decision-making means. Research is presented regarding students' development and application of **experience and intuition in clinical decision-making** during their nursing programme and first year as registered nurses (Standing, 2005, 2007, 2010a). The pros and cons of experience and intuition in nurses' decision-making are then summarised.

What do experience and intuition in decision-making mean?

Experience

In general terms experience refers to anything and everything we have ever thought, felt, sensed or done. In addition to predetermined genetic characteristics, the accumulation of life experiences helps to shape our unique individuality and interests, and the choices we make. Previous experience motivates us to develop knowledge or skills in particular activities, just as Simon did in relation to the case study. Previous experience can influence how receptive we are to, and how we make sense of, the continually changing situations we come across. This is often referred to as 'learning from experience' or 'the university of life'.

Formal education in schools or universities is a highly regulated learning experience focusing on developing thinking skills that are demonstrated and assessed through written examinations. In contrast, learning from life experience is an informal process focusing on combining practical skills, sensory perception, feelings and thinking skills as appropriate to fulfil particular tasks. In nursing education there is a balance between formal, university-based learning and informal, work-based learning. This is because nursing is a practice-based discipline that applies a wide range of thinking, emotional, observational, interpersonal and practical skills to patient care. It is not feasible to develop, apply and integrate all these skills without sufficient clinical experience. For example, the male nurse in the case study understood principles of wound healing (thinking skill), noticed how deeply the arm was lacerated by the broken glass (observational skill), empathised with how young Simon was feeling (emotional skill), communicated with him in a friendly and playful way (interpersonal skill) and demonstrated how to bandage a wound (practical skill).

Hence, with experience, we learn, make connections between, and apply thinking, observational, emotional, interpersonal and practical skills to situations. Each person's experience is unique to them, so it is not easy to 'put our finger' on its exact nature; it is only through experience that we can fully integrate theory and practice in delivering holistic (bio-psycho-social-spiritual) care. Activity 7.2 asks you to test this explanation of experience by applying it to your practice.

Activity 7.2   *Critical thinking*

As nursing is a practical discipline we can be really sure we have learnt useful skills or knowledge only when we apply them in caring for patients. Identify something you have learnt to do as a nurse within clinical practice. Answer the questions below to compare and contrast the skills you applied before and after gaining this practical experience.

1. Describe any nursing activity or procedure you learnt to do as a nurse in clinical practice.
2. Use the format in Table 7.1 to compare and contrast skills used the first time and the last time you performed the activity.

Skills used	First time you did a nursing task – examples of skills used	Last time you did the nursing task – examples of skills used
Thinking Observational Emotional Interpersonal Practical		

Table 7.1: Grid for comparing and contrasting skills

3. Evaluate the effect of experience on your level of competence in using and combining these skills.

As this is for you to review your own experience, no outline answer is given, but you may find it useful to discuss your responses and any related development needs with your clinical mentor.

In completing Activity 7.2 you were asked to do something that may seem slightly unnatural: analysing your experience by relating it to certain criteria (the range of skills). One of the more exciting things about human experience is that it is often spontaneous, unpredictable or even chaotic, and you are never completely sure what is going to happen or how you will react to it. Over-analysing events may therefore seem to miss the point as the true meaning of experience is, arguably, embedded in social contexts and so is only fully understood by participating in them. As mentioned before, studying nursing is not restricted to academic lectures; work-based learning in practice is vitally important for us to become competent nurses. However, we need to develop ways of representing what we do in practice in order to explain or justify decisions and actions, and continually develop a wide range of knowledge and skills. The frequent use of case studies in this book and others in the series helps to portray realistic clinical contexts in which decision-making takes place. Similarly, the activities for readers facilitate learning by asking you to relate the chapter contents to your own clinical experience.

In summary, experience is like an open book of what happens to us throughout our lives, to which we are constantly adding new pages. The contents of the 'book' are so varied and so extensive it is impossible to be fully conscious of everything we have experienced at any one time. For this reason experience is sometimes referred to as tacit, **embodied knowledge**, meaning it is hidden in our mind somewhere like a forgotten memory. To draw on experience in dealing with similar situations we need to somehow 'index the contents' of our 'book' to aid recognition, recall and application of relevant knowledge and skills lying dormant within us. This is why nurses are required to keep personal and professional portfolios of their clinical experiences (see Chapter 8). We also need to be attentive to tacit, **embedded knowledge**, which is concealed within the clinical environment or social context we are interacting with. It is as if the social world is a virtual library full of valuable information cues for us to learn from, which can help to trigger memories of things we have observed before, and may be applicable now. Hence experience informs 'common sense' understanding and decision-making by matching our personal, embodied knowledge to information cues embedded in the social contexts we interact with. The following case study helps to illustrate this point.

Case study: Talking to an unconscious patient

Nancy and Fred are nursing students on practice placement in a medical ward. They are working together to care for Robert, aged 49, who has been unconscious for more than a week. Robert is able to breathe on his own but is otherwise totally dependent on nurses for personal hygiene, pressure area care, intravenous feeding, catheter care, and gentle flexion and stretching of joints in his arms and legs. Fred asks Nancy, 'Do you think he is ever going to wake up?' Nancy replies, 'There is always a chance that he might.' Sister suddenly appears and gives the pair a solemn look before saying very softly to Robert, 'Your wife called to say she will visit this afternoon.' She again looks Nancy straight in the eye and without saying anything more walks away. The pair both feel that sister is non-verbally 'telling them something', and as the more senior (third-year) student, Nancy thinks she should know what it was. Then it 'clicks' as Nancy connects in her mind the way sister spoke directly to Robert, the fact that she and Fred were talking about Robert as if he was not there and being told previously that unconscious patients might still be receptive to sounds (even if they appear unresponsive). She remembers a story about a patient waking up after being in a coma for several weeks during which time his favourite music was played to him, and relatives regularly spoke to him. Nancy follows the sister's lead and says, 'Robert, we are going to give you a wash to freshen you up, and Fred will give you a shave so you look smart when your wife comes to see you.'

Nurses can forget things they have experienced or learnt before. When this happens their actions are not evidence-based and may also be inappropriate. Without 'spelling it out', sister's intervention did enough to challenge Nancy to think more carefully about what she was doing in this particular clinical context. Nancy was then able to piece together the information cues she had missed before, and revise her actions. Sometimes connections are formed subconsciously, which is how experience helps to inform intuition.

Intuition

Intuition refers to a 'sixth sense' or feeling about someone or something or what you should do, without being able to fully explain why or provide any firm evidence to support such 'hunches'. Meeting someone for the first time and making instant judgements about whether you like or dislike, trust or mistrust, or feel safe or unsafe with them, involves exercising intuitive judgement.

We are prompted to use intuitive judgement when:

- we have to make up our mind quickly about something;
- we need to attend to many different things at once;
- we do not have sufficient scientific evidence at hand to inform decisions.

Intuitive judgement is a subconscious process using pattern recognition to make connections between various information cues embedded in a particular context, weighing up what it all means and taking appropriate action (Hammond, 1996). Pattern recognition is a holistic way of thinking developed as we attend to various stimuli or cues in adapting to our surroundings. The male nurse in the first case study used intuitive judgement in making use of the teddy bear (which Simon happened to take along to the hospital with him) to make connections between Simon's young age, physical trauma, anxiety, need for support and play as a medium of communication.

Experience and intuition in decision-making

When newly recruited nursing students were asked to describe their understanding of decision-making, many identified experience as a key component. It included significant life events such as marriage and parenthood, and relevant work experience as healthcare assistants (HCAs). In the next case study a student describes being mistaken for a staff nurse.

Case study: Mistaken for a staff nurse

When asked about her decision-making experience, Serena said she had worked in a mental health unit for two years as an HCA before starting the nursing programme. No uniforms were worn in the unit, which made it more difficult for newcomers to know who was who at first glance. During her last six months there, Serena said two nursing students allocated to the unit, whom she showed around and explained things to, actually thought she was a staff nurse instead of an HCA. It appeared that Serena's experience had enabled her to learn about and explain the organisation and function of the unit beyond that normally expected of the role. To test out Serena's knowledge and understanding of decision-making further, she was asked to imagine meeting a new patient and then describe how she would go about planning care for this person.

continued . . .

Serena replied, 'Hopefully I would have some background notes before I went in so I would read those, sit down, have a chat, find out what she needs from me and then I would go about implementing those to the best of my ability. Assess the whole time because things obviously change. I like to write things down so that I can see how I progress and see if I need to change.'

Serena's response showed she had learnt to take account of different sources of information for assessment purposes and that patient involvement in care planning is important, demonstrating understanding of how plans can be made responsive to the changing needs of patients. She was also aware of the value of recording information and observations for progress monitoring.

The case study indicates what can be learnt in clinical practice to aid understanding of care delivery and organisation (without any formal professional education). It does not mean practical experience is a substitute for theory and research, but it emphasises how knowledge and understanding is also embedded in the clinical environment. Effective clinical decision-making integrates theory and practice in matching principles of evidence-based care to the realities and variations of each patient's unique healthcare needs. Hence, as nurses we are intermediaries between explicit, global scientific research and tacit, local, experiential knowledge in striving to deliver care that is both evidence-based and patient-centred. This is complex and challenging work. Getting the balance right, where relevant research is applied in a way that takes account of patients' personal needs and preferences, requires practice and experience. Experience also complements the use of collaboration (Chapter 2) and observation in decision-making (Chapter 3) as we develop our repertoire of (thinking, practical, observational, emotional and interpersonal) skills in interacting with and monitoring the progress of patients we care for.

As we saw in the case of Nancy and Fred, emulating role models' good practice and learning from our mistakes are also valuable experiences that help enhance decision-making.

Some registered nurses who had recently completed their nursing programme linked greater clinical experience with developing and trusting their intuition to deal with challenging **critical incidents** in caring for patients. It was as though they had developed 'antennae' that sharpened up their receptivity to what was going on around them, understanding the healthcare implications and guiding how they might respond. This supports an increasing association between practical experience and intuitive decision-making as nurses develop from novice, advanced beginner, competent and proficient to expert practitioners (Benner, 1984). For the purposes of this book, experience and intuition in decision-making is defined as follows:

Experience and intuition in decision-making is recognising similarities and differences between current and previous situations and being guided by what seemed effective before (and learning from any earlier mistakes) or realising you lack the necessary experience to make a decision.

Development of experience and intuition in nurses' clinical decision-making

This section presents research describing the development of a group of nursing students experience and intuition in decision-making, over a four-year period (Standing, 2005, 2007, 2010a).

First-year nursing students

Of the 20 students in the research sample, 8 (40 per cent) were aged 17–25 and 12 (60 per cent) were 26–45. Many students therefore had quite a bit of life experience behind them at the start of the nursing programme. All students had some previous healthcare experience, and some had a lot.

- Five had less than one year of healthcare experience.
- Eight had between one and five years.
- Two had between five and ten years.
- Five had over ten years of healthcare experience.

Most of the students had worked as HCAs in nursing homes for the elderly, general hospitals, mental health units or a learning disabilities residential care home. Other experience included foster care for autistic children and voluntary work; helping adolescents with epilepsy; answering a student support helpline. One had worked in an ambulance service control centre for ten years, prioritising emergency calls; one had dispensed medicines at a pharmacy for 11 years; and one had trained as a nurse 20 years before but failed the final exam.

When Simon (in the case study on page 112) was 16 he asked his school for a healthcare placement as a work experience option, mistakenly thinking he would be able to care for people the way he was cared for as a child. Instead, he found himself shaving, washing and toileting elderly men, and this experience discouraged him from studying nursing. However, nine years later (after managing a fast food restaurant) Simon decided he really wanted to be a nurse after all. Other more mature students also felt it was the right time to study nursing now their children were older and less dependent. Parenthood gave them opportunities and experiences in decision-making, as the following case study illustrates.

Case study: Looking after your own child

When asked to give examples of how she made decisions, Clare described how she used her experience to care for her daughter before seeking medical help.

'I had to make an assessment of what was wrong with my daughter. She looked very tired, flushed and unwell, had a sore throat and a bad headache, and complained that the joints in her arms were tender. She lacked energy to do anything, had a high temperature and was "off" her food. It seemed more than just a cold. I thought it might be flu (influenza) as this can sometimes affect the joints.

continued . . .

> *Either way the GP surgery discourages patients from making appointments for such ailments as there is not much they can do, there is a risk of spreading germs and resting at home is often all that is needed to aid recovery. I gave her "over the counter" paracetamol and ibuprofen tablets to relieve pain and swelling and help to lower her temperature, encouraged her to drink lots of fluids and eat what she could, and ensured she had plenty of rest. I got a feeling it was more than flu as she seemed to get a bit better only for the same symptoms to recur again. We decided she needed to see a doctor as whatever she had was beyond me. A physical exam and blood test confirmed glandular fever, which is also a viral infection, so there is no cure for it. The recommended treatment was what I was doing already, but at least we knew what was wrong and why it lasted for so long. The GP said it might take a few months for symptoms to go away.'*

The case study is an example of how newly recruited nursing students had relevant previous decision-making experience in caring for others despite lacking professional education. Activity 7.3 asks you to relate the concept of pattern recognition, discussed earlier, to the case study.

Activity 7.3   *Decision-making*

Earlier it was argued that tacit knowledge and skills (things that are known but are difficult to identify or explain) inform experience and intuition in decision-making. 'Embodied' tacit knowledge is each person's subconscious accumulation of experience, while 'embedded' tacit knowledge refers to information cues in the environment and social context we interact with (Lam, 2000). We combine embodied and embedded knowledge to make sense of situations we find ourselves in. This involves pattern recognition as we make connections between different information cues.

This activity is intended to help you apply the concept of pattern recognition to the case study.

Clare had no professional healthcare education when she assessed and cared for her daughter, so she was not familiar with current evidence-based practice. Instead, she used her experience and intuition to piece together signs and symptoms (information cues), consider alternative causes, make a provisional diagnosis and subsequently question the accuracy of this. Answer the following questions regarding Clare's application of pattern recognition in the case study:

1. Clare thought her daughter's illness was more than a cold, and could be flu. Why did the pattern of signs and symptoms appear to fit flu rather than a common cold?
2. What did Clare notice in the pattern of signs and symptoms that did not seem to fit flu?
3. What pattern of signs and symptoms is actually shared by cold, flu and glandular fever?

Some possible answers can be found at the end of the chapter.

Collectively, the newly recruited nursing students evidently had a reasonable amount of relevant previous decision-making experience. They referred to five of ten perceptions of decision-making discussed in this book (collaborative, systematic, prioritising, experience, confidence) during their first interview (soon after starting the nursing programme). From this point on, theoretical input and practice placements associated with the nursing programme further contributed to their personal understanding, experience and development of clinical decision-making skills.

Second-year students

By now the students had experienced a range of hospital and community practice placements, which extended their understanding of decision-making. This was highlighted by their reference to the other five perceptions of decision-making discussed in this book (observation, standardised, reflective, ethical sensitivity, accountability). Students associated extra clinical experience and patient contact with a chance to develop their competence in performing practical procedures such as dressings, and understanding how medication and other treatments work. They also appreciated opportunities to gain experience in planning care, as the next case study shows.

Case study: 'What about this? What about that?'

Mark recalled how he arranged with his mentor to practise planning care for a patient and how he found being quizzed by the mentor invaluable in getting him to think of things he had overlooked.

'The first care plan I wrote my mentor said, "What about this? What about that?" I didn't think of stuff because of my lack of knowledge and experience. The more experience you have of the outcomes of similar cases the more you are able to make a decision about the best pathway.'

The case study shows how students valued practical experience and mentor support to identify gaps in knowledge and skills, and to develop their decision-making competence in planning care.

Students also experienced times when, due to staffing, equipment or organisational problems, they felt stressed when mentor support was not available.

Case study: Stressful day on the ward

Hazel described a stressful experience in a surgical ward: 'I went on one day, a staff nurse short, extremely busy ward, four people going to surgery who all needed preparation.

- *They had to wear a special gown – we hadn't any of them.*
- *They had to have a special bed-pack – we did not have enough of them.*
- *We had to complete forms – the senior student had not done it before and made errors.*
- *We had to take blood pressure (BP) – the electronic BP machines had broken down.*

I was going to different wards, finding this, finding that. The stress was enormous, and at the end of it I went home feeling terrible about the whole thing.'

The case study illustrates how a shortage of experienced staff and lack of equipment put extra strain on nursing students, trying to compensate for organisational and managerial problems in preparing already anxious patients for major surgery. It was a lesson in how *not* to deliver high quality care and ensure patients have a positive healthcare experience. It also shows how even inexperienced nursing students in practice placement areas may find themselves in situations where they can make a difference. The next case study further illustrates this.

Case study: Preventing an accident

Sally described learning to be alert to unexpected events she might have to respond to or anticipate and prevent threats to patients' safety, if possible, during her practice placements.

'If I felt it was something I could do, I would get on and do it, especially if that person's life was at risk, or if it was a dangerous situation as they might fall or hurt themselves, or something bad that I could stop from happening. I know I'm only a student and I have to report possible problems to a more experienced nurse, but sometimes if you don't act straightaway, a patient is in trouble. On my last placement the floor was being polished. I noticed that as the cleaner went further up the ward the electric lead got caught on a bed and was suspended above the floor. Maude, aged 77, who was short-sighted and a bit deaf, was walking back to her bed at the time and so I just went up and unplugged the polishing machine to make sure she did not trip over the lead.'

The case study shows how clinical environments can be hazardous to patients' wellbeing if nurses and others are not vigilant in continually assessing and controlling health and safety risks. Sally was able to piece together information cues (pattern recognition) in assessing and managing a risk to Maude's safety, realising she might not see the lead and might not hear her warning. Sally's alertness and prompt action may have prevented a fall that could possibly have resulted in a serious injury to Maude. In doing so she was applying activities of living and risk assessment theory to practice in maintaining a safe environment (Roper et al., 2000; HSE, 2011). Activity 7.4 asks you to think about your experience in contributing to and maintaining a safe environment for patients.

Activity 7.4 *Reflection*

Identify examples of risks to patients' health and safety in the clinical environment that you have experienced or witnessed, and describe information cues that suggested patients were at risk. How can you apply what you have learnt from this experience to maintain a safe environment for patients in the future?

As this is for your own reflection, no outline answer is provided.

Third-year students

The next time the nursing students were interviewed they were approaching the end of their nursing programme. They were asked to think about how personal, theoretical and practical influences had contributed to their experience in acquiring and applying clinical decision-making skills. Their responses are summarised in the following three case studies.

Case study: Personal influences on experience and intuition in decision-making

Students identified personal influences as growing up, taking the initiative and 'second nature'.

(i) *Growing up was associated with general life experience outside of the nursing programme, which helped students understand patients' or relatives' concerns: 'Life experience has helped a lot. Since starting the course I left home and got married, and we set up our own home. I feel it has helped me to communicate and empathise with patients' partners better than I could before.' Growing up was also associated with personal development that accompanies observing or participating in challenging clinical situations and being responsible for other people's lives as nurses: 'I've grown up. It's definitely a profession where you mature quickly over three years.'*

(ii) *Taking the initiative was related to a belief that the more you actively participate, the more skills you can develop, and, to seeking out new learning opportunities in the clinical areas: 'I tend to put myself forward to go and experience things on the ward that other people may not.'*

(iii) *Second nature referred to learning to trust your experience and intuition in guiding activities that you have developed skills in, and how 'over analysing' can disrupt performance: 'Once you've had the experience, you go a certain way without thinking about it too much. It's like if you're walking downstairs and you start thinking about where to place your feet, you fall over.'*

The students' ability to identify personal influences in their use of experience and intuition in decision-making supports the idea that becoming a nurse integrates *personal* and professional development. In other words, even academic input has to make sense to students in terms of their own experience otherwise they are unlikely to remember or apply it as they interact with patients. The next case study links theory with experience and intuition in decision-making.

Case study: Theoretical influences on experience and intuition in decision-making

Just as students felt personal influences (growing up, life experience) benefited professional practice, they also applied theoretical influences (research evidence) to their own personal development needs – 'It was really learning to manage my own time effectively to reduce stress levels, then finding a way to de-stress' – and to their relationships with family, friends and others – 'People know that I've been studying to be a nurse. They approach me and quiz me about their health problems, and they expect me to know what the answers are!'

The students' integration of theory and research within their experience of nursing practice was mainly related to the earlier discussion of systematic (Chapter 4) and standardised (Chapter 5)

continued . . .

> decision-making – 'Evidence-based stuff, research, theoretical input about assessment of patients: that, I think, is what most decisions are based on' – and (to be discussed later) reflective (Chapter 8) and ethically sensitive (Chapter 9) clinical decision-making – 'Interpersonal skills, awareness of ourselves, hopefully incorporate into decision-making to avoid making mistakes.'

Being able to relate theory to our personal experience and understanding is important if we are going to apply it in other situations. Similarly, we need to be receptive to and learn from practice placement experiences and apply this to decision-making, as outlined in the next case study.

Case study: Practical influences on experience and intuition in decision-making

The students really valued their practice placements in providing them with many work-based learning opportunities to develop and apply experience and intuition in decision-making, and to:

- *interact with patients, relatives, nurses and others: 'You cannot know how much pain someone is experiencing unless you talk to them, so I asked her to describe it to me'; 'Looked at family's ways of communicating with the patient and added it to care plan'; 'Talking with staff about wound assessments, it's all knowledge that is passed on';*
- *emulate experienced role models and mentors: 'Last mentor is a great role model – she looks at the whole picture but also notices very small things that are relevant'; 'I had an excellent mentor who questioned my judgements, helped to draw things out of me';*
- *develop observation skills of patients' wellbeing: 'Observation is the most important tool; on ward (not hypothetical situations) you base decisions on what you see'; 'Tended to take fluids and supplements in morning, so that was our window of opportunity with patient';*
- *become skilled in performing clinical procedures: 'Gentleman had deep cavity pressure sore, distressed by the smell, dressing had adhered to wound, I needed to use saline to loosen it, I read new dressing should be smaller than wound, so added that to care plan';*
- *assess, plan, deliver and evaluate nursing care: 'If patient off colour, using your head to work out why'; 'Adapted core care plans, added additional things the patient needed';*
- *reflect and learn from practical experience: 'The way we handled situation wasn't right; vowed next time to do it differently' – 'Supervision groups to reflect, listen and learn';*
- *understand nurses' responsibilities and accountability: 'Been given responsibility, child protection issues to deal with'; 'Lowering the level of observation for a mental health patient is a multidisciplinary decision but if we feel person should go to a higher level of observation that's something nurses do to be safe'.*

The examples given by the students indicate they had developed, integrated and applied their thinking, practical, emotional, observational and interpersonal skills in decision-making. This was associated with more in-depth experience and responsibility in interacting with and caring for patients. A hint of intuitive judgement was suggested, but students' decision-making was mainly guided by procedures, guidelines and experienced role models. Activity 7.5 asks you to relate personal, theoretical and practical influences to your experience.

Activity 7.5   *Reflection*

Identify examples of personal, theoretical and practical influences in developing your thinking, practical, emotional, observational and interpersonal skills. Describe how you incorporated these skills in developing and applying experience and intuition in your own decision-making.

As this is for your own reflection, no outline answer is provided.

Activity 7.5 focused on a range of influences in our preparation to become nurses. We now look at what happens once the nursing programme is finished. In the final interview the research sample's experience and intuition in decision-making as registered nurses is described.

First-year registered nurses

The respondents were registered nurses with 6–12 months' experience when interviewed for the last time. Despite having a preceptorship period to get used to their new role, they found the transition from student to staff nurse very challenging, as the following comments suggest.

- *'Responsibility so great so soon.'*
- *'Scary.'*
- *'Accountability nightmare.'*

Their anxiety was associated with an acute sense of responsibility and accountability, and was compounded by a loss of student status or 'comfort blanket' and not being able to 'run for help'.

They also found it a formative period of development, as the following comments show.

- *'Had to learn quickly.'*
- *'Thinking on your feet.'*
- *'Learnt more since qualifying.'*
- *'For that first six months it's a huge learning curve.'*
- *'Boundaries for what you feel comfortable doing shift upwards to more complicated things.'*

It is as if nothing can fully prepare us for 'coming of age' as registered nurses, and there is no substitute for the experience in being personally responsible and professionally accountable for our clinical judgement, decision-making and interventions in caring for others. Several nurses described examples of developing and applying experience and intuition in decision-making in relation to 'reading' patients' body language, feeling 'out of your depth' and assessing patients in emergency situations, as the following case studies illustrate.

Case study: 'Reading' patients' body language

Serena was a staff nurse in a surgical ward where it was the custom to reposition the beds of patients going for surgery (so they could be observed more closely). She noticed that a patient looked worried about what was going on.

Serena said, 'The lady thought that because we moved her there she was on her way to the morgue because the last patient whose bed was moved had actually died. She never said anything – the fear was in her eyes. I could see she was frightened, so I asked, "What's the matter?" I explained, "You were moved because you're a pre-op lady, you can't be too far from the nurses' station as we need to keep an eye on you just to make sure you are all right."'

The case study illustrates that we need to continually check how patients are experiencing the care we provide and to achieve this we need to be observant, perceptive and responsive to any concerns they may have. It also shows how important it is *not* to assume patients understand what is going on but to take time to explain things to them, preferably before they happen. In the next case study it is the nurse who is anxious and unsure of what is going on.

Case study: Feeling out of your depth

Simon (see page 112) was now emulating the nurse who cared for him as a child by working in an emergency care unit. However, when an acutely ill boy was brought in by anxious parents, he felt he lacked the knowledge and skills required to help him.

'The little lad was fitting, and it was important he had this drug (Paraldehyde). I felt really bad at having to say, "I'm not happy giving this" because I was unfamiliar with it, and because it was corrosive (it needed a glass syringe as it could eat through plastic). I asked one of the other staff nurses and she said "No" as she had not given it before either. The only person who could give it was the registrar. I felt quite vindicated that I didn't have blame shoved on my shoulders. It was just a lack of knowledge and fear. I'm not a child nurse, but I have to administer drugs to children. You're so paranoid about it you have to check everything. I went home with the drug information and read up on it in my own time so that next time it happens I am happy to give it.'

Simon knew the boy was acutely ill and needed treatment, and that nurses usually administer medication as prescribed by doctors, but intuitively he felt he was not competent to do it, as shown in Table 7.2.

Experience and intuition is valuable in sensing when we lack the skills to help patients and must, therefore, avoid harming them through our lack of competence. Experience and intuition in decision-making may also apply subconscious insights that can help patients, as the final case study illustrates.

Conceptions of nursing	Experience and intuition in decision-making
Caring	Realising the boy needed specialised skills to care for him.
Listening and being there	Listening to parents' description of son's fitting episode.
Practical procedures	Special type of injection procedure requiring glass syringe due to corrosive nature of the drug (Paraldehyde).
Knowledge and understanding	Lacked knowledge of drug and no experience in giving it – commitment to learn about it for future reference.
Communicating	Asked nursing colleague about her experience of drug.
Patience	Felt vindicated in resisting perceived pressure to give drug.
Teamwork	Sought out team member with necessary expertise.
Paperwork and electronic record	Drug chart, and information sheet about Paraldehyde.
Empathising and non-judgemental	Understood boy would be anxious to get the right help.
Professional	Recognised he lacked competence to safely administer injection so declined, to avoid putting the boy at risk.

Table 7.2: Integrating experience and intuition in decision-making and conceptions of nursing

Case study: Assessing patients in emergency situations

Mark, who had been a staff nurse in A&E for nearly a year, explains his understanding of experience and intuition in decision-making in this highly pressurised clinical context.

'Someone saying, "I've got chest pains" but who looks well and who's observations are normal is going to wait longer than someone complaining of chest pains who is grey, sweaty, pale, short of breath and just looks awful. You start processing those things without really thinking about them.

In fact, because the nursing station has a clear view where the ambulances pull up, as the doors open we sometimes look at what might be wrong with patients and what triage category (scale of urgency from [1] immediate resuscitation to [5] non-urgent) we think they're going to be. Once they're in the department you talk to them and do a full assessment, and sometimes we find we got it right. I think maybe your unease about a patient can come before the exact reasons you're uneasy.

I recently saw the guidelines for calling out the medical emergency team, which include things like pulse and respiration, and the last category was "nurse concern", which they consider equally important. It's a build-up of experience, a kind of unconscious assessment process; you are concerned about a patient but couldn't exactly put your finger on why. That adds to the points score used to decide if a medical emergency team should go to hopefully avert a cardiac arrest.'

Mark's explanation of experience and intuition in decision-making regarding emergency care reflects many of the points made earlier in the chapter. It involves matching our own personal experience (tacit – embodied knowledge), to what we perceive around us (tacit – embedded knowledge) and using pattern recognition to connect and make sense of information cues. Recognising familiar patterns of signs and symptoms in differentiating one condition and level of urgency from others tends to happen subconsciously and more quickly with experience.

In Activity 7.6 you are asked to think about why clinical settings such as emergency care may prompt the use of intuitive judgement and pattern recognition to guide decision-making.

Activity 7.6   *Critical thinking*

As discussed earlier in the chapter, pattern recognition is associated with intuitive judgement and involves making associations between our experience and information cues in our environment. Why do you think emergency care nurses might apply intuitive judgement/pattern recognition?

Some possible answers can be found at the end of the chapter.

Activity 7.6 focused on the use of intuitive judgement. Mark's account of experience and intuition in decision-making also showed how it may complement more scientific evidence-based care as we can check out 'hunches' through observations or investigations of various human functions.

Chapter summary

This chapter attempted to explain what experience and intuition in decision-making means and how it is developed and applied. We looked at knowledge and understanding hidden in our collection of personal experiences (tacit – embodied) and information cues in our environment (tacit – embedded), and how pattern recognition makes connections between them to inform decision-making. We looked in detail at the research study which underpins this book, following a group of nurses throughout their nursing programme and first year as registered nurses, and showing how they applied experience and intuition (Standing, 2005, 2007, 2010a). Case studies demonstrated personal, theoretical and practical influences in developing and applying experience and intuition in decision-making. Strengths of experience and intuition included: being receptive to patients' experience of care; attention to holistic range of information cues in clinical contexts; and being able to make quick decisions. Weaknesses included the following: it is a bit vague and 'woolly'; it may be affected by personal biases; and it may be dismissed as unscientific. So where possible it needs to be tested more systematically. In the next chapter we look at more conscious ways of reviewing experiences, learning from them and applying them to inform reflective judgement in nurses' clinical decision-making.

Activities: brief outline answers

Activity 7.1: Reflection (page 112)

You may have included the following points.

1. Point of bandaging teddy bear: children learn about the world through play, so by bandaging the teddy bear, the male nurse was communicating with Simon at the right level for him to understand about how he needs to protect and take care of his own wound.
2. Impact of male nurse's intervention: it helped turn a trauma into a positive experience of being understood and cared for by balancing seriousness with the right amount of fun to cheer Simon up and reduce anxiety. The experience contributed to Simon's motivation to become a nurse 22 years later.
3. Lessons that might apply to adult care: it highlights the need to combine technical and interpersonal skills; communicate at the right level to ensure mutual understanding and collaborate in patient-centred clinical decision-making; and it gives adults a positive experience of healthcare and enhances their future wellbeing.

Activity 7.3: Decision-making (page 119)

You may have included the following points.

1. Flu more severe, more parts of body can be affected including *joints*.
2. Flu recovery usually within week, recurring symptoms and duration of condition unlike flu.
3. All caused by virus, all have cold symptoms (flu and glandular fever have additional symptoms).

Activity 7.6: Critical thinking (page 127)

You may have included the following points:

*   Intuitive judgement used in A&E as some decisions have to be made very quickly.
*   Pattern recognition used as we need to attend to many things at once, for example, many different patients and having to prioritise who we should attend to first.
*   We may not have the scientific evidence we need to inform more accurate decision-making.

Further reading

Holm, AL and Severinsson, E (2016) A systematic review of intuition: a way of knowing in clinical nursing? *Open Journal of Nursing*, 6: 412–425. Available at: www.researchgate.net/publication/303595322.

Reviews 352 studies linking intuition to patient-centred nursing practice and argues that the development of nurses' intuition is enhanced by maturity, and using intuition increases their sensitivity to patients' needs.

Rovithis, M, Stavropoulou, A and Rikos, N (2015) Evaluation of intuition levels in nursing staff. *Health Science Journal*, 9(3): 4. Available at: www.researchgate.net/publication/282209242.

A single study of 122 nurses working in two hospitals in Greece who responded to a questionnaire designed to assess their use of intuition. It suggests that intuition enhances nurses' emotional and physical awareness, and can help them in developing meaningful connections with their patients.

Chapter 8
Reflective judgement and decision-making

Chapter aims

By the end of this chapter, you should be able to:

* explain how reflection converts experience into learning;
* give examples of reflective judgement and decision-making;

(Continued)

(Continued)

- distinguish between reflective and intuitive decision-making;
- identify personal, theoretical and practical influences on decision-making;
- understand the importance of reflexivity in reflective decision-making;
- consider the pros and cons of reflective decision-making.

Introduction

This chapter looks at reflective judgement and decision-making in clinical practice. As nurses we are expected to reflect on our experiences to learn how to improve care we give to patients (professional development) and learn about ourselves in the process (personal development). This is evident in the NMC *Standards for pre-registration nursing education* (NMC, 2010), which emphasise self-awareness and reflection to convert experience into learning. You may well have been introduced to ways of structuring reflections about your experiences in order to learn from them by applying models of reflective practice (e.g. Gibbs, 1988; Johns, 2010). This is also reinforced by the requirement to keep up-to-date professional portfolios in order to log observations, activities and reflections in our ongoing development as nurses (Reed, 2015). These portfolios are important because they form part of nursing students' assessment, and following registration as nurses they give potential employers an indication of whether our skills match job requirements.

Recording experiences and reflections is also a useful way of researching how nurses develop and apply clinical judgement and decision-making skills. Each decision-making skill identified in this book came from students reflecting on their development in becoming registered nurses (Standing, 2005, 2007, 2010a). Like experience and intuition (Chapter 7), **reflective decision-making** is based on clinical experience. The main difference between intuitive and reflective decision-making is that the former is subconscious and spontaneous while the latter is conscious and deliberate. The following case study helps to illustrate some differences between these two styles.

Case study: Why did I say that?

Second-year nursing students were asked to reflect on their practice placement experiences. They described a range of 'critical incidents' they had been involved in, been affected by and learnt from. Many of these occurred while interacting with patients or relatives where students were less closely supervised than when performing specific clinical procedures. They were, therefore, more self-reliant at these times, judging what to say, or not say, according to their appraisal of the situation and any relevant experience. Heather, a mature nursing student in a surgical unit, was very self-critical when describing how she had responded to a patient.

'A lady waiting to go to surgery said, "My husband died six months ago and it's times like this I really wish he was here and I could say go and get us a cup of tea, love." I didn't think and said, "Oh yes, well thank goodness I have got my husband at home because he would be running around after me."

continued . . .

As soon as I said it I thought, "You stupid woman! Why did I say that? She must have thought what an insensitive thing for me to say." [At this point the interviewer asked Heather to think of an alternative way of responding.] I should have just said, "You must really miss him and for safety reasons we cannot give you a drink before surgery, but when you come back from theatre, and you have recovered from the anaesthetic, we'll make sure you get a cup of tea."

We don't actually know if the lady was upset by Heather's response. Heather was self-critical for answering without thinking, which led her to talk about herself rather than being focused and sensitive to the patient's feelings. She realised her misjudgement straightaway, but the moment had passed and she did not feel able to make amends at the time. Heather's disappointment prompted further reflection, resulting in her identifying a more appropriate response. From this incident she learnt to think more carefully about what she said to patients, to be wary about the appropriateness of unthinking self-disclosure lacking in therapeutic purpose and to value communication skills as nursing interventions.

The case study highlights differences between intuitive and reflective decision-making. Heather intuitively and spontaneously disclosed information about her husband and then with hindsight reflected, reviewed what happened and learnt to respond in a more patient-centred manner. Because intuition is a subconscious process, it is difficult to analyse, so we can only really judge if it is accurate when reviewing outcomes of intuitive decisions. We have no reason to question our intuition if we seem to be getting on well with other people. However, when Heather became aware that she was talking about her own husband, she put herself 'in the lady's shoes' and realised it was an insensitive and unhelpful thing for her to say. Through reflection she learnt to balance rapport, sensitivity to patients and achieving therapeutic goals (e.g. being supportive while indicating it was not a good idea to drink tea before having surgery). Activity 8.1 invites you to use reflection in reviewing an interaction you have had with a patient.

Activity 8.1   *Reflection*

As mentioned above, when we converse with others we tend to draw on our own experiences and sometimes we may not even realise we are doing it. As nurses it is important to develop a good rapport with patients, but it can be tricky to strike the right balance between being friendly and being professional in the way we communicate. Think about the conversations you have had with patients and see if you can recall times when you did not know what to say, or you felt you said the wrong thing, or the patient or relative appeared upset with what you were saying. Then answer the following questions in order to complete your own reflective cycle.

- Describe an incident in as much detail as you can (what happened, when, where, who with).
- Write down how this made you feel and how you think the patient or anyone else involved may have felt (e.g. were you self-critical like Heather was?).

(Continued)

continued . . .

- Identify why you felt the way you did (e.g. Heather was angry with herself because she thought she was 'a stupid woman') and whether you have had similar thoughts or feelings before.
- Describe what, with hindsight, you might have done differently to achieve a better outcome.
- Explain how you might apply lessons from this reflective exercise in your future interactions.
- Test it out next time you find yourself in a similar situation and note whether you feel more self-aware in how you communicate with patients, and if this helps you address their needs.
- Reflect on what you have learnt about balancing skills in establishing rapport, sensitivity to patients and achieving nursing goals. Write up this exercise in your professional portfolio.

As this activity is for your own reflection, no outline answer is provided.

Both the case study and Activity 8.1 reinforce the idea that reflection is valuable in facilitating professional and personal development by converting experience into learning. This can then be applied to inform future clinical judgement, decision-making and nursing interventions. It is often prompted by an awareness that something did not go as well as it should have, which may result in self-denigration (like Heather) or in blaming others. To avoid getting stuck in such negative emotions we need to use these incidents as learning opportunities, work out how we can improve, test it out, review progress and continually develop ourselves as nurses and as people.

This chapter clarifies what reflective judgement and decision-making in nursing is; compares and contrasts intuitive and reflective decision-making; explores ways that reflection can convert experience into useful learning; looks at how reflective decision-making involves integrating personal, theoretical and practice knowledge within an experiential cycle; explains the importance of **reflexivity** to enhance the accuracy of reflective clinical decision-making; and, finally, summarises the pros and cons of reflective judgement and decision-making in nursing.

Reflective judgement and decision-making in nursing

When nursing students were asked about their perceptions of clinical decision-making they described how reflecting on practical experience and interactions with patients helped them to understand and develop their role in contributing to nursing decisions and actions.

> *It is important to be internally reflective. If you don't think about your experiences you don't learn from them, how it has affected you and other people and what you would do differently next time.*

The students found this form of experiential work-based learning very different from the academic input, theory and research they studied at university. In practice placements what they needed to learn was not made explicit in a PowerPoint presentation; it was embedded in the clinical context itself in recognising and addressing patients' constantly changing healthcare needs. One student described how this put more responsibility on her to make sense of things.

You have to put things together in your mind and make connections because the books don't always. You have to be able to work things out for yourself.

Like experience and intuition (Chapter 7), reflective decision-making involves nurses relating personal experience (embodied knowledge) to information cues in clinical practice (embedded knowledge). Getting to know patients enables us to recognise changes in patterns of behaviour, speech or facial expression and the possible healthcare implications, such as recognising when an asthmatic person urgently needs to inhale a drug to dilate their air passages. Through reflection these 'taken for granted' tacit embodied and embedded knowledge and skills can be identified, made more explicit by describing them, and perhaps related to relevant theoretical principles. Table 8.1 summarises the similarities and differences between intuitive and reflective decision-making.

Table 8.1 also illustrates how reflective decision-making involves consciously reviewing experience and taking time to deliberate about what the best course of action is. The delay in decision-making can be relatively short, such as taking a minute to think of what to say when you notice a visitor has given a newly diagnosed diabetic patient a large box of milk chocolates, or it can take much longer, such as judging whether a patient who has been treated for depression after attempting suicide is now well enough to be discharged from an acute mental health unit. Thinking about what action to take when interacting with patients is called reflection-in-action and taking time out to look back at what happened and learn from it is called reflection-on-action (Schön, 1983). In the case study on pages 130–1, Heather was aware she had made a

Focus of comparison	Intuitive decision-making	Reflective decision-making
Main source of information	Practical experience	Practical experience
How information processed	Pattern recognition	Pattern recognition
Use of nursing knowledge	Tacit (embodied, embedded)	Make tacit knowledge explicit
Level of mental awareness	Subconscious	Conscious
Speed of decision-making	Immediate	Delayed
Type of decision-making	Spontaneous	Deliberate
Explaining decision-making	Felt it was right at the time	Describe personal rationale
Auditing quality of decisions	Patient outcomes	Rationale and patient outcomes

Table 8.1: Comparing and contrasting intuitive versus reflective decision-making

mistake when talking to the lady waiting to go to surgery but was unable to think of an alternative intervention at that time. Looking back at the incident she was able to think of a better response through her reflection-on-action.

The practice-based nature of reflective decision-making therefore complements experience and intuition (Chapter 7), observation (Chapter 3) and collaborative decision-making (Chapter 2) for nursing care to be patient-centred and relevant to patients' needs and preferences. The ability to explain one's reasons for decisions and how they are intended to benefit patients also means that the process of reflective decision-making is auditable. This is important for professional accountability as nurses *must practise in line with the best available evidence* (NMC, 2015, p7). Whereas evidence-based practice is usually associated with applying research through systematic (Chapter 4) and standardised (Chapter 5) decision-making, nurses' observations and reflections can often provide valuable evidence to support best practice (Ellis, 2016). This is strengthened where nurses can demonstrate working through different steps of a reflective cycle, just as you did when reflecting on interacting with patients in Activity 8.1. For the purposes of this book:

Reflective decision-making is understood to mean a conscious and deliberate process informed by learning from previous experience, which has a 'personal rationale' that can be explained to others. It involves pausing for thought to review events as they occur (reflection-in-action) and choose the best nursing option or to review past events (reflection-on-action) and help to inform future practice.

Using reflection to convert experience into useful learning

We can use reflection to review and learn from our experiences individually, with someone else, or in group situations. In the following case study Jo, a second-year nursing student, describes her own private way of disentangling what has happened in the clinical area in order to 'unwind' and relax when she goes home.

Case study: Thinking things through in the shower

'When I get home from a shift I would be straight in the shower and think about things: Why did I do that? What led to it? Should it have happened? If I was there again, having hindsight, would I do it that way?

I think it through in the shower, which is my thinking space, and when I come out I leave it behind because if we kept everything with us continually and thought about it 24 hours a day we would all go loopy, but I could spend 45 minutes in the shower contemplating things.'

A lot can happen during a shift and there may not be time to 'take it all in', which poses questions or 'food for thought' for when there is more time to reflect on events. Jo found working through her own reflective cycle – to make sense of her experience in clinical practice – necessary and beneficial in order to disengage from work ('leave it behind') when she got out of the shower. If she did not create space for reflection, Jo suggests she would remain stressed ('go loopy') as things might continue to nag her. Jo uses the ritual of showering (washing the cares of the day away) in a very positive way to aid her reflection. Hence, there may be occupational health benefits for nurses and other health professionals to have opportunities for reflection. It also contributes to lifelong learning and professional development, as indicated by Jo in casting a critical eye on what she might do to improve her effectiveness as a nurse. Activity 8.2 asks you to critically review the value of individual reflection as described by Jo.

Activity 8.2   *Critical thinking*

Do you, like Jo, have your own individual way of reflecting back on what has happened in clinical practice? What do you think are the strengths and weaknesses of using individual reflection to convert experience into useful learning?

Some possible answers can be found at the end of the chapter.

Sometimes it may be easier to reflect on incidents when discussing them with someone else, such as a friend, colleague or mentor. In the first case study Heather was still 'stuck' at being angry with herself until she was asked to think of an alternative response, which helped her to 'move on'. In Chapter 4, nursing students acknowledged how being questioned by their mentors helped them to identify things they had not thought of before when planning systematic care. Supportive and challenging mentoring and supervision in nursing can, therefore, facilitate the development of clinical competence in reflective decision-making (Standing, 1999). Activity 8.3 asks you to think about how you might discuss your reflections with someone else.

Activity 8.3   *Communication*

Have you shared your thoughts and feelings in reflecting on clinical experience with another person? What 'ground rules' do you think are important to adhere to for this to be effective? How might reflecting with someone else be more or less effective than reflecting on your own?

Some possible answers can be found at the end of the chapter.

As we saw in Chapter 2, many clinical decisions are collaborative, involving contributions from different healthcare professionals, as described by one of the students.

Decisions on the ward are normally part of a multidisciplinary thing, rather than just one individual saying, 'This is how it's going to be', because others will bring different insights to the situation. So, by having more of you, you can get a better approach.

It seems sensible, then, to have opportunities for team members to reflect on events together, as needed. In the following case study Clare, a second-year nursing student in a children's unit, recalls her first experience of group reflection and the benefits she associated with it.

Case study: Talking it through

'We had a terrible day on my placement: a baby died first thing; we had a horrendous non-accidental injury; and then a GP sent in a child with leukaemia. The nice part was at the end of the shift everyone sat down and talked about it. The doctors were there as well. I had never seen that before, and although I didn't have much input I didn't feel the need because I was listening to what the team had to say. The importance of reflection was really brought home to me that day. It did actually prompt me to look more at the child protection issue.'

Any one of these events is challenging to deal with, but all three occurring together during the same shift must have been extremely demanding both emotionally and professionally. The death of a baby is a tragic loss for the parents, and can affect nurses and other team members, too, while they are also trying to be sensitive to the parents' grief. A non-accidental injury is disturbing because it is usually caused by adults entrusted with the care of the child, and the healthcare team have a legal responsibility under the Children Act 1989 to report it immediately to social services, to ensure the child is protected from further abuse. On top of this, the team needed to care for a newly admitted seriously ill child who was suffering from leukaemia (cancer of the white blood cells).

Despite feeling 'out of her depth' Clare was positive about it because she had participated in an inter-professional support group, which was a unique and productive experience for her. The team appeared to recognise that too much had happened for nurses, doctors and others to leave the unit without reflecting on the events in a supportive atmosphere. This type of reflection was not just checking whether the right decisions and actions had been taken; it also enabled staff to express their feelings about the traumatic events in a non-judgemental manner. Being sensitive to each other's need to de-stress can help health professionals be more sensitive to patients because they feel less overwhelmed by their own emotional baggage. Acknowledging and ventilating emotions (catharsis) can also help to 'clear the mind', enabling nurses and others to develop deeper understanding and focus on what they need to do (Heron, 2001). Witnessing the above events and listening to her colleagues helped Clare to value reflection. This prompted her to fill a gap in her own knowledge regarding child protection policy and procedures, and nurses' responsibilities in applying them. In Activity 8.4 you are asked to think about participating and reflecting on your practice in an inter-professional support group.

Activity 8.4   *Team working*

Have you had any experience of contributing to healthcare team discussions or participating in supportive, therapeutic or supervisory group work? How might group reflection by a healthcare team remove or reinforce barriers to effective inter-professional teamwork and decision-making?

Some possible answers can be found at the end of the chapter.

This concludes our look at the different ways of converting experience into useful learning by reflecting on practice individually, in pairs or in groups. In the next section we look at the range of knowledge and skills that are developed, integrated and applied in reflective decision-making.

Integrating personal, theoretical and practical influences

Becoming a nurse involves both personal and professional (theoretical and practical) development. As a nursing student you begin the programme with a unique personal history and outlook, and all the theory, research and work-based learning you experience are filtered through and interpreted by your own values and expectations. The further you progress through the programme the more opportunities there are to integrate increasing amounts of theoretical and practical knowledge in your personal experience of becoming a nurse. Reflection is a means to connect and integrate personal, theoretical and practical worlds. Mark, a second-year student, reflects on his professional development.

Case study: Satisfying to teach a procedure

'The new experience of being a student on the wards was quite difficult to enjoy at first because you felt incredibly useless, so when people were busy there was very little I could do. I enjoy my placements much more now that I have got more competent in certain practical skills. I've come to value the clinical skills that I have been learning more than perhaps I did at the start. I was focusing more on the person-to-person aspect then. I get self-esteem from being caring, someone the patients get on with, but also from being able to do technical things that perhaps they don't understand. I have found it very satisfying to teach a procedure to a student nurse (who was earlier on in the programme than me), that I had a skill they didn't have that I could impart to them.'

Like many nurses, Mark appears to get personal satisfaction from being useful in helping to care for patients. This ambition was initially frustrated by his lack of knowledge and skills, but then he developed competence in practical skills to a level that he could teach more junior students.

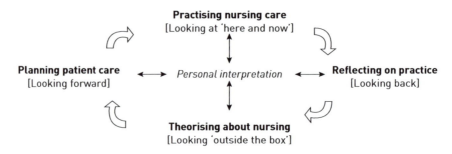

Figure 8.1: Reflective decision-making: a personal/practical/theoretical/experiential cycle

The technical nature of some skills also required a theoretical understanding to fully appreciate their use and purpose. Figure 8.1 summarises how personal, practical and theoretical influences are integrated in an ongoing experiential learning cycle (adapted from Kolb, 1984 and Standing, 2005, 2007, 2010a) where reflection has a key role in making sense of experience, and shaping future decisions and interventions.

In Figure 8.1 the most important stage of the cycle is practising nursing care, but in order to ensure that this is well-informed and continually adjusted to be relevant in addressing patients' changing circumstances, the other stages of the cycle are also needed. The various perceptions of decision-making discussed in this book complement some elements of the experiential cycle more than others, as shown in Table 8.2. Ultimately, nurses' judgement and decision-making are personal choices for which they are professionally accountable. This is why personal interpretation lies at the heart of this adapted experiential cycle, both influencing and influenced by each of the stages. Identifying how the students interpreted their experiential learning was elicited using hermeneutic phenomenological research methods which promote collaborative exploration of the respondents' and the researcher's inter-subjective understanding (Standing, 2009).

The experiential model of reflective decision-making is strongly grounded in and matched to holistic patient-centred care and clinical contexts in which it is delivered. It requires nurses to apply a range of thinking, practical, emotional, interpersonal and observational skills, including, but not limited to, theory and scientific research where relevant to patient care. This holistic view of reflective decision-making is supported by multiple intelligences theory (Gardner, 1983), which identifies linguistic, logical–mathematical, spatial–visual, bodily–kinaesthetic, musical–auditory,

Elements of the experiential cycle	Perceptions of decision-making
Practising nursing care	Experience and intuition, Collaborative
Reflecting on practice	Reflective, Observation
Theorising about nursing	Ethical sensitivity, Prioritising
Planning patient care	Systematic, Standardised
Personal interpretation	Confidence, Accountability

Table 8.2: Elements of the experiential cycle and perceptions of decision-making

inter-personal and intra-personal forms of intelligence, complementing the above range of skills. Logical–mathematical intelligence is the most analytical form, and is usually associated with scientific and theoretical concepts. As such, it links with 'Theorising about nursing' in Figure 8.1 and supports critical thinking associated with reflexivity in decision-making.

Reflexivity in reflective decision-making

This chapter has made a case for the importance of reflective decision-making in nursing, but it can be open to criticism for potential personal bias or misinterpreting information cues. There may be a greater danger of this where nurses are reflecting individually rather than in pairs or groups. It is not always possible to test out our interpretation of events or proposed actions with others and, in any event, we are individually accountable for our decisions. It is therefore wise to find a way of self-monitoring our judgement and decision-making for possible inaccuracies. This means assuming that our interpretations could be wrong, finding ways to test them and being open about our potential biases. Researchers call it reflexivity, which basically means critically examining the way we reflect on our experience and interpret observations. When applied to clinical decision-making, reflexivity has been defined as follows:

> *Lifelong learning in the critical self-examination of ideas, assumptions, biases and any lack of knowledge or understanding that may impede sound patient-centred clinical judgement and decision-making, plus a commitment to take action and improve knowledge and skills.*
> (Standing and Standing, 2010, p214)

Applying reflexivity in reflective decision-making is particularly important in order to accurately assess serious health risks. We will look at two case studies using critical incidents (events having a significant impact, prompting us to reflect and learn from them) with contrasting outcomes.

Case study: I was angry with myself

Mark has been a staff nurse in an A&E unit for nearly a year. One day Derek, aged 35, is admitted because he has become confused. He is accompanied by his wife. Mark assesses Derek, not knowing he had been in a car accident 24 hours before and had sustained a head injury. Derek is too confused to mention it, and his wife does not either because he had a skull X-ray in another hospital and they didn't find anything wrong. Derek has suffered a brain haemorrhage and dies within a couple of hours. Mark blames himself for not considering the possibility that Derek's symptoms were caused by a head injury.

'I was very angry with myself. I'd made an assumption and continued down that route until it was forcibly thrust to my attention something was very wrong. When I'm working in A&E I can get influenced by paramedics' assumptions, and that's "tripped me up" a couple of times. If a paramedic has a preconception that a patient is faking it, I have to work very hard not to think the same. It's not the nursing role to make a medical diagnosis, but we have to pick an appropriate category to do the triage (prioritise most urgent cases). From that incident I learnt to be:

(Continued)

continued . . .

- *less fixed in what I think;*
- *less dependent on what other people think;*
- *more ready to make my own decisions.*

Initially I learnt the wrong lessons. The next day another patient was unwell, and we didn't know why.

He was in the same cubicle and was my responsibility. I was very anxious and wanted a doctor to see him immediately. The doctor had a quick look and said he'd be all right – it was probably just a transient ischaemic attack (temporary lack of oxygen to the brain) – the same provisional diagnosis I had incorrectly attributed to Derek. I was getting upset. I had to take off and say to myself, "Calm down, it's not the same patient, it just feels the same", because I felt sure if I didn't get help immediately he was going to die as well.'

The case study highlights the life-and-death nature of many nursing decisions, the fine line between these possible outcomes and how making errors can shake confidence. In doing so it conveys some limitations of reflective decision-making in that it depends on the quality of available information such as identifying an accurate history of the onset of a patient's illness and current symptoms. Unreliable witnesses who are not forthcoming with relevant information or make inaccurate assumptions can cloud your judgement. Relying upon observation and reflection to the exclusion of more scientific evidence may result in relevant research being ignored. From this incident Mark learnt to be reflexive in evaluating opinions and advice he received (*less dependent on what other people think*), to think for himself (*make my own decisions*) and acknowledge the tentative nature of his decisions (*learnt to be less fixed in what I think*). Activity 8.5 invites you to explore the concept of reflexivity in more depth.

Activity 8.5   *Evidence-based practice and research*

Do an online literature search on the concept of reflexivity, including qualitative research in which it is often applied to demonstrate control of researcher bias. Devise your own working definition of reflexivity that you can apply in critiquing the accuracy of your reflective decision-making. With reference to your definition, develop a couple of questions that can test your reflexivity.

As this is for your own personal research, no outline answer is provided.

In the previous case study Mark's reflexivity swung from being underdeveloped when he was unaware of the seriousness of Derek's condition to being overdeveloped after Derek died, when he no longer trusted his powers of observation and reflection. The change was influenced by Mark's emotional distress in failing to detect the head injury and being unable to save Derek's life. This illustrates how stressful registered nurses' decision-making responsibilities can be. It reinforces the point made earlier about the need to talk about traumatic events in a supportive setting, and highlights the need for reflexivity to reduce bias and inaccuracy in decision-making.

In the next case study, a staff nurse is faced with an emergency she does not feel experienced enough to deal with, but she is the only nurse present.

Case study: He's not breathing

Clare recalled a mother approaching her suddenly, in a state of distress.

'The lady shouted, "He's blue, he's not breathing!" and threw this baby into my arms. There wasn't anyone with me, no one in shouting distance. I was shocked by the urgency of a situation I was not prepared for, but something in the back of my mind helped me to assess, realise this child had an obstruction in his airway and realise that I needed to clear it immediately. I laid him face down on my lap and patted his back four times, he coughed, some thick mucus came up, and he started breathing again and changed back to his natural colour. If I hadn't been taught what to look for, I wouldn't have been able to do it. I just pictured [Nurse Tutor] explaining what to look for in a child with severe respiratory distress and what to do. Afterwards we had a reflective talk on the unit and it was nice to know I had done everything the senior member of staff would have done.'

The critical nature of the baby's condition and the absence of immediate support meant that Clare found she was alone with the responsibility of reviving the baby, with a very anxious mother in attendance. She managed to remain sufficiently composed in these challenging circumstances, and in the absence of relevant previous practical experience, dealt with the emergency. Clare's ability to understand what was wrong and what she needed to do about it involved 'reflection-in-action', matching her observations of the baby to a recollection of a lecture and video at university regarding identifying and relieving an obstructed airway in a baby. Clare did not actually feel competent to deal with the emergency. If a more experienced person had been present, she would have deferred to them, but the baby was blue and had stopped breathing. If she had gone looking for someone else to help, it might have been too late to save him, so although she had not done it before, she felt she had to try to revive the baby. Table 8.3 shows how Clare integrated reflective decision-making with conceptions of nursing.

In linking the conceptions of nursing to Clare's reflective decision-making, Table 8.3 also shows that Clare successfully applied the '6Cs' (care, compassion, competence, communication, courage, commitment) advocated by health policy (DH, 2012a). We can also apply the reflective decision-making experiential cycle (Figure 8.1), showing how Clare integrated personal/theoretical/practical knowledge and skills, plus the other perceptions of clinical decision-making described in this book.

Conceptions of nursing	Reflective clinical decision-making
Caring	Doing everything possible to help the baby breathe.
Listening and being there	Being attentive and responsive to the mother's cry for help.
Practical procedures	Using an approved method to unblock the airway.
Knowledge and understanding	Linking the baby's appearance with respiratory distress.
Communicating	Trying not to show how worried she was.
Patience	Not panicking when confronted by the emergency.
Teamwork	Reflecting and receiving supportive supervision after the incident.
Paperwork and electronic record	Recording what happened in the nursing records.
Empathising and non-judgemental	Understanding how distressing it was for the mother and baby.
Professional	Carrying out effective risk assessment and management of the emergency.

Table 8.3: Integrating reflective clinical decision-making and conceptions of nursing

- *Practising nursing care (Looking at the 'here and now')* – Clare was receptive to the mother's 'cry for help' about her baby not breathing (*Collaborative*) and knew this was a very serious situation but one that she had no experience of dealing with (*Experience and intuition*).
- *Reflecting on practice (Looking back)* – Clare could see that the baby had turned blue and was unable to breathe (*Observation*). She realised something had to be done quickly to enable the baby to breathe, that she was the only nurse present and that there was no time to find an experienced nurse (*Reflection*).
- *Theorising about nursing (Looking 'outside the box')* – Clare linked the baby's breathing problem to a lecture she remembered on airway obstruction and what to do to clear the airway (*Prioritising*). Clare had a dilemma because she was not supposed to carry out procedures that she was not competent in without supervision, but if she didn't, the baby might die (*Ethical sensitivity*).
- *Planning nursing care (Looking forward)* – Clare understood that the baby probably had something stuck in the airway that needed removing to resolve the problem and restore normal breathing (*Systematic*). She visualised the technique she had seen on a video accompanying the lecture on how to position the baby and apply a sequence of pats to the back (*Standardised*).
- *Personal interpretation* – Clare felt very anxious at first and 'out of her depth' but tried not to show it as the mother was already distressed (*Confidence*). The baby needed urgent care, and she was the only nurse present, so Clare performed the procedure as best she could despite her inexperience (*Accountability*). In implementing her plan ('Practising nursing care' in a continuing cycle of reflective decision-making), Clare achieved a successful outcome that justified her actions and boosted her confidence.

As mentioned in Chapter 1 and demonstrated in the above discussion, nurses' decisions involve all of the perceptions of decision-making presented in this book. Collectively they portray a comprehensive overview of clinical decision-making in nursing. We have also seen that reflective decision-making is a vital part of this process in recognising where there is a health problem and in formulating a way to resolve it.

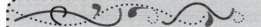

Chapter summary

This chapter presented different aspects of knowledge and understanding in nurses' reflective decision-making. For example, we explored the concepts of embodied and embedded knowledge, which were related to personal and professional development in converting clinical experience into useful learning through reflection-in-action and reflection-on-action, privately, in pairs or in groups. The patient- and practice-centred basis of reflective decision-making was compared and contrasted with experience and intuition in decision-making. It was argued that reflection helps to articulate personal and practical knowledge that remains hidden in intuitive decision-making. An experiential, reflective decision-making model was proposed, integrating personal, theoretical and practical influences and associated thinking, practical, emotional, interpersonal and observational skills. This closely complements the principles of holistic nursing care. Examples and case studies of reflective decision-making in different pathways from junior nursing student to registered nurse were provided, together with a variety of activities to help readers relate theory to practice. The strengths of reflective decision-making include: its relevance to patient-centred care; its recognition of the importance of information cues and observations in the clinical context; and its contribution to 'grass roots' nursing knowledge and expertise. The weaknesses include: its local focus, which might mean it ignores relevant national research that could benefit patients; the fact that it is limited by the quality of observations and available information cues; and the potential for bias and inaccuracy by decision makers when interpreting experience. It was argued that the concept of reflexivity, borrowed from qualitative research, is a valuable process to raise awareness and help control personal bias by critically examining and testing out our assumptions wherever possible.

Activities: brief outline answers

Activity 8.2: Critical thinking (page 135)

You may have included the following points.

Strengths:

- Time and place of one's choosing.
- As often as you like.
- Privacy and peace.
- Autonomy – self-care.

Weaknesses:

- Limited perspective.
- Support not available.
- Views unchallenged.

Activity 8.3: Communication (page 135)

You may have included the following points.

Ground rules:

- Agree aims.
- Clarify roles.
- Confidentiality clause.

Pair more or less effective than individual?

- Dependent on both adhering to agreed ground rules.
- Less effective if collusion occurs.
- More effective if trusting, honest, supportive and challenging.

Activity 8.4: Team working (page 137)

You may have included the following points.

Remove barriers:

- Group perceived to be relevant by team members.
- Opportunities for interaction and mutual understanding.
- Possibly enhance effectiveness of integrated care pathways.
- Identifying, valuing and pursuing shared objectives.

Reinforce barriers:

- No consensus about perceived need for group.
- Group members do not have equal status.
- Used to criticise or embarrass colleagues.
- No values or objectives shared by group.

Further reading

Gallagher, S and Payne, H (2015) The role of embodiment and intersubjectivity in clinical reasoning. *Body, Movement and Dance in Psychotherapy*, 10(1): 68–78.

Philosophical discussion reflecting on how to share understanding of embodied personal, practical and experiential knowledge in order to inform valid psychotherapeutic decision-making in mental healthcare.

Howatson-Jones, L (2016) *Reflective practice in nursing* (3rd edn). London: Sage/Learning Matters.

Many interesting case studies of learning through reflection in different areas of nursing practice.

Chapter 9
Ethical sensitivity in decision-making

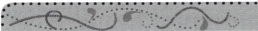
Chapter aims

By the end of this chapter, you should be able to:

- explain ethical sensitivity in nurses' decision-making;
- identify and apply ethical principles to nursing practice;
- relate the NMC *Code* to nurses' duties in decision-making;
- discuss topical ethical issues and dilemmas in nursing;
- appreciate that ethical values affect all nursing decisions.

Introduction

This chapter discusses **ethical sensitivity in decision-making**. As nurses we are duty bound to abide by a professional and ethical code (NMC, 2015) at all times, so each decision we make has to be ethically justifiable. Ethical sensitivity in decision-making involves applying moral values and ethical principles in caring for patients, their families and the general public.

For the purposes of this chapter the following understanding of the term is adopted:

> *Ethical sensitivity in decision-making is applying ethical principles (patients' freedom of choice, actions should benefit not harm them, and fairness to all) in respecting patients' dignity and confidentiality, enabling their informed consent, and resolving moral dilemmas in nursing care.*

In this chapter we explore the theory and practice of ethical sensitivity in decision-making by:

- discussing and applying relevant RCN principles of nursing practice;
- exploring the philosophical basis and influence on clinical decision-making of different ethical theories;
- summarising ethical principles in healthcare and relating them to the *The Code* (NMC, 2015);
- outlining how moral and ethical considerations are incorporated in law.

Case studies and learning activities highlighting ethical issues and dilemmas when caring for patients help to link theory and practice throughout the chapter. Finally, the strengths and weaknesses of ethical sensitivity in nurses' clinical decision-making are summarised.

Ethical sensitivity in RCN principles of nursing practice

The Royal College of Nursing has identified eight principles (A–H) of nursing practice to guide nurses in how to apply robust ethical and professional values in caring for patients (RCN, 2010). In this chapter we will refer to these principles of nursing practice, which flag up ethical issues such as enabling a person to die peacefully and with dignity. It is especially challenging and heart-rending when the dying patient is a child, as illustrated by the following case study. The dignity, bravery and maturity of the young child in the case study is remarkable, and in the first five learning activities in this chapter you will be asked to reflect on the ethical sensitivity shown in her care.

Case study: 10 going on 80

Habib, an interpreter, is reflecting upon his involvement in the care of Yasmin, a terminally ill 10-year-old girl whose family immigrated to the UK from Pakistan. Habib's main role is to enable communication between Yasmin, her family and the doctors and nurses. In this particular instance his role is to convey Yasmin's last wishes to her father. Habib explains that Yasmin has received

continued . . .

medical treatment for most of her young life. She is very small for her age, almost blind and partially deaf; she has poor control of her bowels, and her kidneys are failing. Habib describes Yasmin as '10 going on 80' as she seems to have such a wise head on such young shoulders in living her severely restricted life to the full, inspiring admiration and respect from everyone who knows her, and in facing up to the inevitability of her own premature death.

Yasmin is cared for in a hospital unit. One day she creates an opportunity to talk to Habib in private by asking her dad to fetch her some clothes, and while he's away she asks Habib to sit down as she needs to ask him something. Yasmin explains she knows she is going to die soon, and when that happens she would like Habib to tell her dad she wants to be buried in Pakistan, next to her grandfather and with all her toys as she doesn't want anyone else to play with them. She says it is difficult for her to talk directly to her dad about this. About a week later Yasmin's health deteriorates and she whispers to Habib to remind him of her request. Sometime later Yasmin dies. Habib tells her dad what she has said. He replies, 'I was going to do that anyway, I loved her'.

(Adapted from RCN video clip illustrating how to apply nursing principles)

Although Habib is not a nurse, his role as an interpreter gives him temporary membership of the healthcare team and also of Yasmin's extended family, both of which are concerned with caring for her. Habib responds to Yasmin's request in a way we as nurses might, and this is why the case study helps to illustrate the following RCN principles of nursing practice.

Principle A

Nurses and nursing staff treat everyone in their care with dignity and humanity – they understand their individual needs, show compassion and sensitivity, and provide care that respects all people equally.

Principle D

Nurses and nursing staff provide and promote care that puts people at the centre, involves patients, service users, their families and their carers in decisions and helps them make informed choices about their treatment and care.

(RCN, 2010, p1)

Now you have read the case study and principles A and D, you are ready to tackle Activity 9.1.

Activity 9.1   *Evidence-based practice and research*

This activity encourages you to look more closely at the evidence presented in the case study. See if you can identify examples where Habib appeared to apply principles A and D (or not). Do you agree or disagree that Habib demonstrated effective application of the principles? Please explain the reasons for your judgement using examples from the case study.

Some possible answers are included at the end of the chapter.

In undertaking Activity 9.1, you make a start at probing and understanding how ethical considerations are part and parcel of everyday healthcare interventions. In RCN principles A and D, the references to dignity, humanity, compassion, sensitivity, respect, equality, patient-centred care and informed choice reflect the application of moral values and ethical sensitivity in nurses' judgement and decision-making. It involves:

- translating caring qualities associated with nurses into clinical decisions and subsequent actions that are humane and professionally competent;
- empowering patients to be active participants;
- achieving the best possible care outcomes.

Maintaining confidentiality, dealing with patients' or relatives' complaints and reporting nurses' concerns about standards of care also involve applying moral values and ethical sensitivity in decision-making. This point is supported by another of the RCN principles.

Principle E

Nurses and nursing staff are at the heart of the communication process: they assess, record and report on treatment and care, handle information sensitively and confidentially, deal with complaints effectively, and are conscientious in reporting the things they are concerned about.
(RCN, 2010, p1)

In Activity 9.2 you are asked to relate RCN principle E to Habib's decision-making in the case study.

Activity 9.2   *Decision-making*

Principle E is applicable to the case study since Habib was *at the heart of the communication process* regarding Yasmin's care, he appeared to *handle information sensitively* when Yasmin effectively told him her 'last will and testament', and he treated this information *confidentially* and only disclosed the details to Yasmin's dad after her death, as she had requested. In order to dig deeper at ethical issues regarding Habib's decision-making, please answer the following.

1. If you were in Habib's place, would you have acted in the same way or not? Please explain why you would/would not or suggest what else you might have done.
2. Do you think Habib was right to keep Yasmin's wishes confidential until after she died as she had requested? If so, why? If not, why not?
3. If someone argues that Habib's actions were wrong because they might encourage vulnerable young girls to share secrets with unrelated grown men, how would you respond to this?

continued . . .

4. Given that when Habib told Yasmin's dad how she wanted to be buried, he said he was going to do that anyway, did Habib actually achieve anything by telling him? If so, what?

5. Imagine Habib is on leave when Yasmin dies and her dad does not know what she said. Now suppose he buries her in the UK, not Pakistan, so he can visit her more often. What potential ethical issues arise from this situation, and how could they have been avoided?

Some possible answers can be found at the end of the chapter.

Activity 9.2 gives you a taste of how to question, defend or perhaps amend decision-making in relation to its possible ethical justification. In order to understand and explain ethical issues in more depth it is helpful to look at relevant philosophical perspectives.

Philosophical basis of ethical sensitivity in decision-making

Philosophy is an advanced type of critical thinking that seeks answers to questions about the meaning of human existence, nature of knowledge, moral values, political organisation and desirable behaviour. The study of ethics is a branch of philosophy, and different philosophers emphasise the importance of different priorities in ethical theory, as briefly outlined in Table 9.1.

Virtues

Aristotle focused on the importance of people developing a virtuous character, which he thought led to personal wisdom, happiness and a strong community. He named it 'Nicomachean' ethics after his son Nicomachus. This helps to demonstrate that developing good character is a consequence of practising the right habits through lifelong learning with input from role models such as parents, teachers and scholars.

Despite being over 2000 years old, Aristotle's focus on human virtues remains very influential: nursing students, like registered nurses, have to demonstrate that they are of good character; for example, a criminal conviction prevents you from becoming or remaining a practising nurse. If you look at the Essential Skills Clusters box at the start of the chapter you can see each one begins with *People can trust a newly registered graduate nurse*. Honesty and trustworthiness are human virtues like those Aristotle associated with ethical conduct. Evaluating appropriateness of behaviour according to whether a reasonable person would have acted similarly in the same situation (Table 9.1) is still used as a guide to dispense legal and moral justice. In Activity 9.2, question 1 invited you to test this out by putting yourself in Habib's shoes and deciding whether or not you would have acted in the same way. Courage, one of

Ethical focus	Virtues	Rights and duties	Outcomes
Defining morality	Being a good person	Doing good things	Getting good results
Examples applying ethical priorities	Honesty, caring, fair-minded, brave	Get informed consent before treating patient	Healthcare problem is satisfactorily resolved
Questioning and evaluating conduct	Would a reasonable person act the same way in the situation?	Did the nurse act in accordance with NMC code of conduct?	Do benefits of care outweigh the costs to patient or to society?
Corresponding ethical theories	Nicomachean (how to develop a good character)	Deontology (theoretical principles of moral duties)	Consequentialism and utilitarianism (maximising benefits)
Philosopher linked to ethical theory	Aristotle (384–322 BC)	Immanuel Kant (1724–1804)	Jeremy Bentham (1748–1832)

Table 9.1: Virtues, rights and duties, and outcomes in ethical theories

the '6Cs' of compassionate care (DH, 2012a), or bravery is another useful virtue for nurses to possess to cope with physical, emotional and mental demands that many people might find difficult. The case study also showed that we can often learn a lot from patients in this respect, given Yasmin's remarkable fortitude in suffering serious illness most of her short life, and facing her fears about dying with such dignity.

Rights and duties

Good personal qualities and virtues such as caring are essential in nursing, but more concrete and specific guidance is needed in applying ethical principles to policies, procedures and decision-making. This is where Kant's deontological theory comes into play since we need to know what patients' rights are so we can make it our duty to respect those rights in our dealings with them. They are referred to in the NMC *Standards for pre-registration nursing education* (2010) under 'professional values', for example, *empower [people to make] choices that promote self-care and safety* (first box, start of chapter). It is reinforced in the Essential Skills Clusters (second box, start of chapter), for example: *empowering people to make choices; gain their consent … prior to any intervention; seeks consent prior to sharing confidential information;* and *people's rights in decision-making and consent will be respected and upheld*. Professional and ethical principles in nursing (NMC, 2015) can also be used to both guide and evaluate nurses' conduct (Table 9.1). In investigating any complaints about registered nurses a panel appointed by the NMC will also refer to *The Code* in deciding whether it has been breached, and whether the nurse remains fit to practise or not (discussed further in Chapter 10, 'Accountability for nursing decisions').

In the case study Yasmin appeared empowered, taking the initiative to ask Habib to convey her burial wishes to her dad after she died. It is unlikely Yasmin would have done this unless she trusted Habib, and he honoured that trust by telling her dad what she said. Activity 9.2 asked you to think about potential ethical implications of Habib keeping his agreement with Yasmin confidential until the time came to reveal what she said. It helps to show that ethical dilemmas can occur where seemingly opposing duties (empowering self-determination of patients while safeguarding vulnerable minors) need addressing. Resolving dilemmas is a judgement call, and it is advisable to involve other healthcare team members (not doing so leaves the practitioner vulnerable to accusations if something goes wrong). If a child is involved, we would normally include parents, but in this case it was against Yasmin's wishes, as she did not feel the time was right for her dad to know what she was thinking about. We do not know whether or not Habib discussed Yasmin's wishes with the healthcare team before he told her dad. Activity 9.2 assumes he did not, whereas Activity 9.3 assumes that he tried to.

Activity 9.3   *Team working*

However good a rapport we have established with a patient, we are part of a team with whom responsibility for care is shared. Communicating significant developments to members of the team is therefore important in order for care to be well informed, responsive to changes, co-ordinated and consistent. This activity asks you to imagine that Habib wants to get Yasmin's consent for him to share her wishes with the team. Please answer the following questions.

1. What are the advantages of sharing the information with the healthcare team?
2. What anxieties might Yasmin have about agreeing to this?
3. If you were in Habib's place, what would you say to inform Yasmin's decision in consenting or not consenting to sharing with the team information she had told you in confidence?
4. If Yasmin is in agreement, what duty of care would team members have in this respect?
5. If Yasmin does not consent to sharing information with the team, what would you do?

Some possible answers can be found at the end of the chapter.

Outcomes

Being of good character, respecting patients' rights and fulfilling our professional duties may contribute to good outcomes of care, but ultimately the success of care is judged by whether the patient's health improves, deteriorates or does not change. Working towards achieving good outcomes for patients is also referred to in the following RCN principle of nursing practice.

Principle G

Nurses and nursing staff work closely with their own team and with other professionals, making sure patients' care is co-ordinated, is of a high standard and has the best possible outcome.
(RCN, 2010, p1)

This is where ethical theories of consequentialism or utilitarianism are relevant since they focus on outcomes. NMC professional values (see the box at the start of the chapter) apply them to underline the importance of achieving outcomes that assure patients' safety while they *manage risk and promote health and wellbeing*. Hence, both consequentialism and utilitarianism emphasise that actions are morally good if the outcomes indicate that things have improved (Table 9.1).

Conversely, actions are morally suspect if things get worse (even if the correct procedures have been followed). This approach can be described as the 'ends justifying the means', which is in direct contrast to rights and duties, which focus more on following the correct procedures or the 'means justifying the ends'. The main difference between consequentialism and utilitarianism is that the latter asserts that outcomes that benefit the greatest number of people are better than those that benefit one or two people. Utilitarianism may therefore be used to link ethics with social theory, politics and economics (e.g. funding more cost-effective treatments so that more people can benefit, while rationing less cost-effective treatments). Activity 9.4 will help you to clarify the differences between these two 'outcomes-focused' ethical theories.

Activity 9.4   *Reflection*

Read the following moral assumptions regarding Yasmin's care. Do you think they are describing the application of consequentialism or utilitarianism? Explain why.

1. It is wrong in today's day and age – with all the medical and scientific knowledge at our disposal – that more was not done to prolong Yasmin's life (we are not told why a kidney transplant that might have enabled her to survive longer was not performed).
2. It is wrong in today's financial climate that so many resources were used to fight a losing battle in keeping Yasmin alive for so long when the money could have saved many more lives by tackling preventable causes of death, for example by increasing the uptake of immunisations against childhood diseases and supervising children at risk of non-accidental injuries.
3. It is right that the healthcare team helped Yasmin to gain a few more years of life (which she truly appreciated and made the most of) than she would have had without their help.
4. It is right that the healthcare team helped Yasmin to gain a few more years of life because in doing so they learnt more about her disease and how to treat it, so the knowledge and expertise will be invaluable in contributing to more effective care of other similar children.

Some possible answers can be found at the end of the chapter.

Activity 9.4 looked at alternative perspectives of whether outcomes of Yasmin's medical care were successful or unsuccessful. In Activity 9.2, you explored the outcomes of Habib conveying or not conveying Yasmin's wishes to her dad as promised. In Activity 9.5 you are asked to apply consequentialism and utilitarianism to Habib's actions.

Activity 9.5   *Reflection*

Read the following moral assumptions regarding Habib's actions and identify whether you think they are describing the application of consequentialism or utilitarianism. Explain why:

1. Habib was wrong not to tell the healthcare team about Yasmin's request because if anything had happened to him, no one else could have told her dad what she said.
2. Habib was wrong not to tell the healthcare team about Yasmin's request because they needed to know what was worrying her to be sensitive to her needs in the last weeks of her life, and also to inform their understanding and care of other children in the future.
3. Habib was right to agree to Yasmin's request because it helped ease her fears about dying to think she would have all her toys with her and be buried next to her grandfather, and it saved her from talking about it with her dad, which she did not feel able to do.
4. Habib was right to agree to Yasmin's request because it not only benefited her, it also comforted her dad and family to know they were doing what she wanted, and, in telling Yasmin's story, Habib helped many nurses value ethical sensitivity in decision-making.

Some possible answers can be found at the end of the chapter.

Both Activity 9.4 and Activity 9.5 highlight the debatable nature of the rights and wrongs of actions and their consequences. In other words, ethical decisions are never 'cut and dried'; there is always an element of uncertainty in wondering whether the right decision has been made, and this makes them the most challenging decisions healthcare professionals have to deal with. Outcomes of healthcare can be interpreted differently as right or wrong, according to the moral assumptions or ethical perspective that is applied. As a general rule of thumb, when we are focusing on getting the best outcomes for a particular patient we are applying consequentialism, and when we are focusing on the bigger picture in getting the best outcomes for all potential patients and the public at large we are applying utilitarianism.

In this section we have used relevant moral philosophy to describe personal qualities (virtues), theoretical principles (rights and duties) and practical benefits (outcomes) associated with ethical sensitivity in clinical decision-making. As nurses we have to combine and apply all of these different strands to be the best person that we can be, provide the best care possible and achieve the best results for patients. In the next section we explore some of the challenges in applying ethical principles and the NMC *Code* in delivering high standards of care to patients.

Applying ethical principles and *The Code* in decision-making

The Code (NMC, 2015) specifies the professional and ethical requirements to practise as a registered nurse. Many of these reflect aspects of moral philosophy and associated ethical principles discussed earlier. If you find the theory a bit difficult to grasp, you do not have to worry too much because as long as you abide by *The Code* you will be applying ethical principles to practice. Four key ethical principles have been derived from moral philosophy, and these are thought to capture the essential virtues, rights and duties, and outcomes that, as nurses, we should always strive to achieve in caring for patients. The four ethical principles are *autonomy, non-maleficence, beneficence* and *justice* (Beauchamp and Childress, 1989). Table 9.2 cross-references them with relevant extracts of *The Code* to help link ethical theory to practice.

Ethical principles	Relevant extracts: *The Code* (NMC, 2015)
AUTONOMY Respect people's right of self-determination and freedom of choice	• *Treat people as individuals and uphold their dignity* (p4) • *Listen to people and respond to their preferences and concerns* (p4) • *Encourage and empower people to share decisions about their treatment and care* (p5) • *Act in the best interests of people at all times* (p5) • *Respect people's right to privacy and confidentiality* (p6) • *Respond to any complaints made against you professionally* (p18)
NON-MALEFICENCE Do not cause people harm (first principle of first aid)	• *Recognise and work within the limits of your competence* (p11) • *Be open and candid with all service users about all aspects of care and treatment, including when any mistakes or harm have taken place* (p11) • *Act without delay if you believe that there is a risk to patient safety or public protection* (p12) • *Raise concerns immediately if you believe a person is vulnerable or at risk and needs extra support and protection* (p13) • *Be aware of, and reduce as far as possible, any potential for harm associated with your practice* (p14)
BENEFICENCE Enable people to achieve best possible state of health and sense of wellbeing	• *Make sure that people's physical, social and psychological needs are assessed and responded to* (p5) • *Always practise in line with the best available evidence* (p7) • *Communicate clearly* (p7), *Work co-operatively* (p8) • *Share your skills, knowledge and experience for the benefit of people receiving care and your colleagues* (p8) • *Keep clear and accurate records relevant to your practice* (p9) • *Be accountable for your decisions to delegate tasks and duties to other people* (p10) • *Always offer help if an emergency arises in your practice setting or elsewhere* (p12)

	• *Advise on, prescribe, supply, dispense or administer medicines within the limits of your training and competence, the law, our guidance and other relevant policies, guidance and regulations* (p13) • *Provide leadership to make sure people's wellbeing is protected and to improve their experiences of the healthcare system* (p18)
JUSTICE Be fair-minded, treat people equally in matching care delivery to their respective needs	• *Avoid making assumptions and recognise diversity and individual choice* (p4) • *Act as an advocate for the vulnerable, challenging poor practice and discriminatory attitudes and behaviour relating to their care* (p5) • *Keep to all relevant laws about mental capacity that apply in the country in which you are practising, and make sure that the rights and best interests of those who lack capacity are still at the centre of the decision-making process* (p6) • *Take reasonable steps to respond to people's language and communication needs, providing, wherever possible, assistance to those who need help to communicate their own or other people's needs* (p7) • *Use range of verbal and non-verbal communication methods, and consider cultural sensitivities, to better understand and respond to people's personal and health needs* (p7) • *Act with honesty and integrity at all times, treating people fairly and without discrimination, bullying or harassment* (p15)

Table 9.2: Autonomy, non-maleficence, beneficence, justice and The Code

Autonomy and beneficence

The principle of autonomy or self-determination underpins Orem's self-care model (Chapter 1) where nurses continually assess what patients can or cannot do for themselves and help them with the latter (beneficence). It is also intrinsic to collaborative clinical decision-making (Chapter 2) where patients actively participate in and influence the nursing decisions that affect them. In the following case study a well-informed, articulate patient is unable to persuade a nurse of the seriousness of her symptoms, and this contributes to the ensuing fatal consequences.

> ### Case study: Fobbed off
>
> *One weekend Miranda, aged 26, woke up with swelling and pain in her calf. She waited until Thursday to see if it would go away. When it did not, she looked at the NHS Choices website (**www.nhs.org.uk**) and entered 'pain in calf' in the 'search' box. It indicated she might have a blood clot – deep vein thrombosis (DVT) – in her calf. Miranda contacted her GP surgery but the earliest appointment offered was for the*
>
> *(Continued)*

continued . . .

following Monday (four days' time). Miranda was concerned about the delay in seeing the GP. She was anxious because she remembered her mum had a DVT at the age of 21 and she thought this might increase her risk of having one. She also took contraceptive pills that increased her risk of blood clots. Miranda took aspirin both for the pain and because she knew it was supposed to help thin the blood.

On Friday, Miranda was so worried about her leg that she attended an NHS walk-in centre where she explained her concerns to Judy, an experienced nurse. Judy did not agree with Miranda's view and advised her to go home and rest as it was probably a muscle strain. Afterwards, she cried as she spoke to her husband on the phone, telling him she'd been 'fobbed off'. Miranda did not see her GP on the Monday because on the Sunday she collapsed and died from a pulmonary embolism (blood clot in the lung), a known fatal complication associated with having an underlying DVT.

(Adapted from 'Woman dies after being "fobbed off"' by Chris Brooke, *Daily Mail*, 20 October 2010)

The case study is a disturbing account of what can happen when a service user's autonomy is disregarded. Through her resourcefulness and intelligence Miranda managed to piece things together and come up with the correct provisional diagnosis. All she needed was a healthcare professional to emulate what she had done (or refer her to someone who could) so that she could receive the right investigations and treatment. Tragically, this was not to be. There are many aspects of the case study that go beyond the scope of this chapter: Was the NHS website advice appropriate? Why couldn't the GP see her sooner? How far away was the main Accident and Emergency centre? We will focus here on Miranda's contact with Judy, the nurse at the NHS walk-in centre.

Activity 9.6   *Leadership and management*

Imagine that you are a lay member on a clinical governance committee at the NHS Trust where Miranda died. Your job is to represent the interests of service users. You are concerned about Judy's inability to do an accurate risk assessment. This has implications for better supervision and continuing professional development of all nurses. You decide to read *The Code* (NMC, 2015) to see what registered nurses are supposed to do. You identify requirements that, had they been complied with, would have meant that Judy might have acted differently, with a better outcome for Miranda.

Please read through the case study and the NMC extracts associated with autonomy and beneficence in Table 9.2 once again, before answering the following questions.

1. Which NMC requirements of registered nurses to respect or empower patient autonomy appeared to be lacking or needing improvement in the case study and why?
2. Which NMC requirements of registered nurses to apply beneficence within high quality patient care appeared to be lacking or needing improvement in the case study and why?
3. What recommendations would you make to improve the NHS Trust's walk-in service?

Some possible answers can be found at the end of the chapter.

Activity 9.6 highlights the importance of registered nurses reading and practising *The Code* in order to effectively apply the ethical principles of autonomy and beneficence. In the next case study a district nurse offers an elderly lady a higher level of care than she actually wants.

Case study: Choosing to live alone

Margaret, aged 81, is a widow who lives alone in a council flat where she has lived for 35 years. Ten years ago she had a stroke, leaving her blind in one eye and with muscle weakness. She also has arthritis, late onset diabetes and difficulty controlling her bladder. Margaret takes tablets for arthritis, blood pressure and diabetes, and wears a pad in case of 'accidents'. She is visited regularly by three daughters who cook for her and ensure she has the right diet. Margaret lives on the fourth floor and there is no lift. She has not been out of her flat for six years since her son-in-law – who used to help carry her up and down the stairs – had to stop after having a heart attack.

Elizabeth, a district nurse, has known Margaret since she had the stroke and over the years has co-ordinated the supply of a walking frame and adaptations in the flat to help her get around, including a sit-in bath, a raised toilet seat, hand rails in the corridor, a stair lift in the short stairway from the living area to bedrooms and an emergency buzzer system she can call for help with. Her family also bought a special armchair that electronically helps her to sit, elevate feet and stand up. Margaret's mobility has deteriorated recently and she has had a number of falls. Her daughters ask Elizabeth to assess Margaret's safety as they believe she now needs constant care and supervision. When Elizabeth sees Margaret she explains that it is possible for her to move to a residential home nearby where she will be looked after on the ground floor so she can get out in the garden (she loves flowers and has lots of pots on her balcony) and the girls can visit as they do now. She tells Margaret that the GP has said he would be happy to support such a referral, and it seems that her daughters believe this is the safest and best thing for her also. Margaret tells Elizabeth she does not want to move, that she loves her flat, and that when the time comes she wants 'to die in my own home'. Elizabeth accepts Margaret's decision and increases her visits to monitor her health and to help Margaret exercise and strengthen her legs.

In this case study, Elizabeth appears to be well aware of the health risks and how these can be controlled, while also respecting Margaret's preferences. In Activity 9.7 you are asked to consider how she was able to achieve this.

Activity 9.7 — *Decision-making*

With reference to the case study and relevant NMC extracts (in Table 9.2), describe how Elizabeth balanced and applied the ethical principles of autonomy and beneficence in Margaret's care.

1. Following Margaret's stroke.
2. In responding to her daughters' request for an urgent assessment.
3. When Margaret declined the residential care option.

Some possible answers can be found at the end of the chapter.

Activity 9.7 highlights a constant tension between respecting someone's freedom of choice and providing the best possible care. Ethical sensitivity in decision-making is therefore challenging, and requires the integration and application of a range of relevant knowledge skills and attitudes. Table 9.3 illustrates this regarding the care Elizabeth provided for Margaret.

Conceptions of nursing	Ethical sensitivity in decision-making
Caring	Committing to maximising Margaret's health and wellbeing.
Listening and being there	Responding to daughters' worries and Margaret's wishes.
Practical procedures	Providing exercises to increase strength/flexibility of Margaret's legs.
Knowledge and understanding	Understanding risks posed by medical problems and Margaret's frailty.
Communicating	Explaining to Margaret possible benefits of residential care.
Patience	Allowing Margaret time to decide what she wants to do.
Teamwork	Liaising with GP/council/social services to get flat adapted.
Paperwork and electronic record	Writing up risk assessment, recommendations and action.
Empathising and non-judgemental	Understanding Margaret's reluctance to move out of her flat.
Professional	Applying NMC *Code* to treat Margaret with dignity and respect.

Table 9.3: Integrating ethical sensitivity in decision-making and conceptions of nursing

Table 9.3 also shows how the conceptions of nursing complement application of ethical principles (autonomy and beneficence) in decision-making. Beneficence and non-maleficence are 'opposite sides of the same coin', the former maximising helpful, the latter minimising harmful outcomes of nursing care. In practice many healthcare interventions, while being helpful, can also have less helpful or sometimes harmful outcomes; for example, antibiotics save lives most of the time, but if someone is allergic to them, they can be life-threatening. It is vital to make sure that benefits of care outweigh costs to each patient's health and wellbeing. Applying non-maleficence requires vigilance in order to avoid making costly mistakes through carelessness or ignorance. This is why in first aid training you are first taught not to harm the victim. This may seem obvious, but if you do not know what you are doing, it can often do more harm than good.

Non-maleficence and justice

Ethical principles of non-maleficence and justice often go together in healthcare because it is unfair for service users to be harmed rather than helped by those they trust to take care of them. One of the areas nurses have to be particularly careful about is the administration of medicines, including checking if it is the right drug, right dose, right route, right person, right time. This is especially important in caring for young children, who need much smaller doses than adults. In the next case study the nurses do not follow procedure properly, with fatal consequences.

Case study: Tragic outcome of misreading prescription

Max was born prematurely, weighing less than two pounds. He needed intensive treatment in a high dependency neonatal unit to enable him to survive. After three months he weighed over six pounds and was thought strong enough to undergo necessary abdominal surgery. Sometime after the operation Max was prescribed an intravenous solution of 5 ml of sodium chloride in 1 litre of fluid to ensure he was adequately hydrated and to maintain the correct sodium level. Instead of 5 ml the ward manager and the staff nurse checking and administering the solution put in 50 ml (ten times the prescribed dose) of sodium chloride by mistake. The overdose led to Max being severely dehydrated. He lost weight, suffered brain damage and died when he was only four months old.

(Adapted from 'First picture of baby who died after suspected salt overdose from hospital drip' by Caroline Grant, *Daily Mail*, 24 July 2009)

The case study graphically demonstrates the importance of vigilance in giving medicines and the danger of complacency in not carefully reading and checking prescriptions. The 'failsafe' system failed. The nurse whose role it was to check what the other was doing should have spotted the discrepancy between what was prescribed and what was being administered and acted promptly to stop her colleague (see 'Non-maleficence' NMC extracts in Table 9.2). All the good work the neonatal unit had done was undone by two nurses' lack of vigilance, with tragic results. It underlines the earlier point that a nurse's first duty is not to harm patients. In Activity 9.8 you are asked to reflect on the implications of the case study in your own area of practice.

Activity 9.8   *Reflection*

As a nursing student you will be asked to help administer medication, including checking if it is the right drug/dose/route for the right patient. You cannot do this safely and effectively unless you understand what the drugs are for, their optimal therapeutic dose, side effects and possible contraindications (people who should avoid them, for example, allergic reaction to antibiotics). Think about the medicines patients receive in your current or previous practice placement and look up the ones you are unsure of (use the current version of the *British National Formulary*). Try to make connections between each patient's health problems and their prescribed medicine so that you know why the patient needs it, how it works and what to watch out for. Do not forget to consider each patient's body weight and how that might affect the prescribed dosage, especially in relation to children. This can help to make what might otherwise seem a routine task more meaningful, and by prompting you to question what you are doing it also helps to reduce errors.

As this is for your own reflection, there is no outline answer provided.

Activity 9.8 and the previous case study suggest that although nurses' first instinct may be to do things to help people (beneficence), they need to counterbalance this by continually assessing health risks they may pose to patients themselves and reducing these (non-maleficence). Sometimes harm suffered by patients is more psychological than physical, resulting from stereotyping, prejudice or a lack of understanding, as the next case study illustrates.

Case study: A patient wants to smoke

Joanne, a third-year nursing student, was reflecting on an incident that occurred during her last practice placement in an acute medical ward. Katia, aged 25, an Estonian tourist visiting London, had collapsed and been admitted to Joanne's ward for observation and investigation. Katia had regained consciousness, but she spoke very little English and communication was difficult. She had an intravenous infusion in her arm to aid hydration. No one knew exactly what was wrong with her because the results of blood tests and other investigations were not yet known. Some HCAs said she was a 'manipulative patient' because she talked 'in her own language', kept wanting to go out of the ward for a cigarette and pulled her intravenous infusion out when no one helped her carry it outside so that she could have a smoke. When the staff nurse saw what Katia had done she shouted at her, and then Katia threw a jug of water at the staff nurse. Joanne thought that Katia was confused, frightened and frustrated that she had no one she could talk to. By the end of the day Katia was transferred to the mental health unit where it was felt they would be better able to manage her 'violent behaviour'.

The case study suggests that nurses and HCAs may not always be as caring, non-judgemental and empathising as the conceptions of nursing (in Table 9.3) advocate. It also highlights an underlying power imbalance in relationships between healthcare workers and service users. In order to guard against this we are expected to empower patients to be active contributors in deciding what's best for them collaboratively (Chapter 2). In the case study the communication problems clearly made this more of a challenge. Katia may have perceived the healthcare team to be uncaring/threatening, and they in turn may have felt that Katia was being unco-operative/hostile and not caring for herself by insisting on smoking and removing the intravenous infusion. These perceptions led to a stalemate of non-collaboration, and because of the underlying power imbalance the healthcare team's view of Katia prevailed and she was removed from the clinical area. Activity 9.9 asks you to apply the ethical principle of justice in reviewing what happened in the case study.

Activity 9.9   *Communication*

Many of the difficulties described in the case study arose from a lack of communication between Katia and the ward staff. Refer to the relevant NMC extracts associated with the ethical principle of justice in Table 9.2 when answering the following questions.

continued . . .

1. Which of the NMC requirements were not addressed in the treatment of Katia?
2. Was it fair or unfair for the HCAs to refer to Katia as a 'manipulative patient'?
3. What could the staff have done to facilitate better communication with Katia?
4. Was it fair or unfair to call Katia 'violent' and move her to a mental health unit?
5. In what way did Joanne differ from her colleagues in her assessment of Katia?

Some possible answers can be found at the end of the chapter.

Activity 9.9 and the previous case study focus on the ethical principle of justice or fairness. Just as we are duty bound to avoid harming patients (non-maleficence), we are also obligated to address biases, stereotypes and prejudices that can lead us to treat others unfairly. Until we can achieve this we will never be able to treat all people fairly or as equals. It is not easy to achieve if nurses are stressed, and the extra demands required by some patients may exacerbate this, leaving them feeling 'burnt out' and unable to cope. An increase in violence against nurses and other healthcare staff in Accident and Emergency centres can compound perceived stress and highlight that nurses also need to be protected. Ultimately, justice is dispensed through legislation, and in the final section we look briefly at how respecting and addressing moral and ethical principles are, in fact, a legal obligation.

How moral and ethical considerations in healthcare are incorporated in law

The virtues, rights and duties, and outcomes we discussed earlier are not confined to texts on moral philosophy. Similarly, ethical principles of autonomy, non-maleficence, beneficence and justice are not confined to university lecture theatres. Throughout the chapter, with reference to topical case studies, we have shown how these ideas can help to distinguish between good and poor nursing practice to maximise the former and minimise the latter. These principles are not confined to nursing, as they are incorporated within British and European law as basic human rights and duties that everyone is both entitled to and bound to abide by. The impetus for this came in the wake of revelations about atrocities in the Second World War. People in the UK are therefore protected by the Human Rights Act 1998, which reflects each of the ethical principles (shown in brackets) that we discussed earlier:

*   *The right to life* (beneficence).
*   *Freedom from torture and degrading treatment* (non-maleficence).
*   *The right to liberty* (autonomy).
*   *The right to respect for private and family life* (autonomy).
*   *Freedom of thought, conscience and religion, and freedom to express your beliefs* (autonomy).
*   *The right not to be discriminated against in respect of these rights and freedoms* (justice).

In order to demonstrate compliance with the Human Rights Act in the UK, the Department of Health set out a framework for applying 'FREDA' (Fairness, Respect, Equality, Dignity, Autonomy) principles and commissioned a human rights healthcare project to research how to do this (DH, 2008b). The resulting human rights based approach recommended for service providers is summarised as 'PANEL':

- **P** = Participation of service users in exercising their right to make decisions about their care.
- **A** = Accountability of service providers in respecting service users' right to receive quality care.
- **N** = Non-discrimination to eliminate any form of discrimination and embrace equality and diversity.
- **E** = Empowerment of service users to know their rights and to participate in having their rights met.
- **L** = Legality of service providers in complying with the requirements of the Human Rights Act 1998.

Mersey Care who provide specialist learning disability services is one of the NHS Trusts involved in the human rights healthcare project. They demonstrated pioneering and innovative ways of applying 'PANEL' principles. Service users including patients and their relatives were asked to contribute to policy making and operational management (alongside service managers and staff representatives) for which they were paid £12 an hour, and treated as equals in the decision-making process. This included their participation on the NHS Trust Board, recruitment and selection of staff, overseeing new service developments and evaluating healthcare provision through the service users' research evaluation ('SURE') group (Dyer, 2015).

It is surprising that learning disability patients, particularly vulnerable to social exclusion, discrimination and abuse, were empowered to participate so comprehensively in the organisation, planning, delivery and evaluation of the healthcare services they use. This does not mean that the rights of liberty or autonomy are not sometimes compromised in order to protect service users from harming themselves, harming others or being harmed by others. The important thing here is that actions taken must be necessary and proportionate for the limited time they are needed, rather than being excessive, punitive or degrading. Staff at Mersey Care reported having a better understanding of service users' needs as a result of the human rights project, and the service users who participated felt their mental health had improved through being involved. It remains to be seen whether other NHS Trusts emulate Mersey Care in showing how ethical sensitivity in decision-making, 'FREDA' principles (incorporated in the NHS Constitution) and compliance with the Human Rights Act can be facilitated in organising, delivering and evaluating healthcare services (DH, 2013a; Dyer, 2015).

Chapter summary

In this chapter we defined ethical sensitivity in decision-making and explored its origins and applications. We identified ethical values in the RCN's principles of nursing practice and explored their philosophical basis in terms of being a good person, doing good things and achieving good outcomes. Four key ethical principles were identified – autonomy,

continued . . .

non-maleficence, beneficence and justice – and they were cross-referenced to relevant extracts of the NMC *Code*. It was noted that ethical principles and moral values are applied within the Human Rights Act 1998 which healthcare professionals and organisations have a legal duty to comply with, and that this is reflected in the NHS Constitution (see Chapter 10). Case studies showed how ethical principles can be applied to examine all aspects of nursing practice, including examples of decision-making that demonstrated ethical sensitivity, and decision-making that lacked ethical sensitivity. A power imbalance between nurses and patients was referred to. Good practice was associated with respecting patients' autonomy and empowering their collaborative decision-making. Poor practice was associated with harming patients, non-collaboration, not respecting patients' autonomy and with unfair treatment. The ethical principles were related to the conceptions of nursing identified in previous chapters, showing how they complement one another. The strengths of ethical sensitivity in decision-making are that it translates nurses' caring qualities into humane, professionally competent interventions that empower patients to be active participants and achieve the best possible care outcomes. The weaknesses of ethical sensitivity in decision-making are that it can be very complex, protracted and contentious because ethical dilemmas are difficult to resolve to everybody's satisfaction. Various activities invited you to grapple with these issues in relation to questions raised in real-life, poignant case studies, to help you to make links between ethical theory and compassionate practice.

Activities: brief outline answers

Activity 9.1: Evidence-based practice and research (page 147)

You may have included the following points.

Applying Principle A (dignity, humanity, compassion): Habib respected Yasmin's courage and wisdom for one so young (10 going on 80) and was sensitive regarding her wishes. His interpreter role helped the family communicate with staff.

Applying Principle D (involve service users, families in decisions): Habib followed Yasmin's lead in discussing her preferred burial arrangements and when to tell her dad about her decision, so, in effect, he allowed the service user to make use of him.

Was Habib successful in applying Principle A and D? Yes, because Yasmin appeared to trust him and he honoured that trust as outlined above.

Activity 9.2: Decision-making (pages 148–9)

You may have included the following points.

1. Say yes if you would do the same as Habib in order to ease Yasmin's fear about dying.
2. Say yes if Habib was right to keep it confidential until the time came, as that was Yasmin's wish.
3. Ordinarily it is unwise to encourage such secrets, but the circumstances were not ordinary. Yasmin initiated it, not Habib, and the reasons for not telling her dad yet were understandable.
4. Habib fulfilled his duty to Yasmin by telling her dad, and he learnt her wishes would be met.
5. The potential ethical consequences would be Habib not honouring his promise to Yasmin. It could have been avoided if he asked to be contacted or if he asked someone else to tell her dad.

Activity 9.3: Team working (page 151)

You may have included the following points.

1. Improved communication, shared responsibility, back-up system if Habib not available.
2. Yasmin may not know them so well, and might be worried they might tell her dad before the agreed time.
3. Sharing information lessens risk of Yasmin's dad not knowing her wishes if Habib is away.
4. Team members' duty of care to respect Yasmin's wishes about when to talk to her dad.
5. If Yasmin does not consent, respect her wishes but make note in reflective journal or diary.

Activity 9.4: Reflection (page 152)

You may have included the following points.

1. Consequentialism – unable to save Yasmin's life.
2. Utilitarianism – unable to use money to save many other children's lives.
3. Consequentialism – managed to help Yasmin gain a few more years of life.
4. Utilitarianism – healthcare team gained knowledge they can use to treat other children.

Activity 9.5: Reflection (page 153)

You may have included the following points.

1. Consequentialism – by not telling the team they could not fulfil Yasmin's wish if Habib was away.
2. Utilitarianism – not telling the team limited understanding so less well informed in caring for others.
3. Consequentialism – eased Yasmin's fears, saving her from talking to her dad about her death.
4. Utilitarianism – Yasmin's story can help nurses apply ethical sensitivity with other patients.

Activity 9.6: Leadership and management (page 156)

You may have included the following points.

1. (i) Listen to people and respond to their preferences and concerns; (ii) encourage and empower people to share decisions about their treatment and care (autonomy), need improving.
2. (i) Miranda's physical, social and psychological needs were not properly assessed or responded to by Judy; (ii) Judy did not practise in line with the best available evidence; (iii) and Judy did not demonstrate leadership to protect Miranda's wellbeing or to improve her experience of the healthcare system.
3. *Recommendations*: Ensure nurses working in all emergency settings have the knowledge and skills to carry out accurate risk assessments; review management and supervision of walk-in centre personnel; ensure nurses are familiar with the NMC *Code* and how to apply it within the specific clinical contexts in which they are practising; when patient refers to NHS website information, use computer to check through information and advice with them.

Activity 9.7: Decision-making (page 157)

You may have included the following points.

1. Arranged for walking aid and adaptations to flat to help Margaret adjust to reduced vision and mobility; gave advice on medication and diet re diabetes; helped her to keep her home.
2. Undertook risk assessment regarding Margaret's frequent falls and deteriorating health; identified supervised residential care option and presented it to Margaret for her to decide.
3. Accepted Margaret's decision to decline residential care and increased home visits to give additional support and help her exercise and strengthen her legs.

Activity 9.9: Communication (pages 160–1)

You may have included the following points.

1. NMC justice requirements not met: (i) staff made unfair assumptions about Katia and did not appear to value diversity and individual choice; (ii) poor practice and discriminatory attitudes were not challenged; (iii) reasonable steps were not taken to respond to Katia's language and communication needs; (iv) staff did not use a range of verbal and non-verbal communication methods, or consider cultural sensitivities, to better understand or respond to Katia's personal and health needs; (v) Katia was not treated fairly without discrimination, bullying or harassment.
2. Unfair for HCAs to call Katia a 'manipulative patient' since they could not understand a word she spoke and could not, therefore, make that judgement unless it was based on prejudice.
3. Enable better communication by contacting interpreter, look up English–Estonian dictionary on the internet, give non-verbal gestures of support (smile) and avoid shouting at her.
4. Unfair for Katia to be labelled as 'violent' and moved to a mental health unit since the team have not managed to communicate with her to make an assessment of her mental health. It was wrong for her to throw the jug, but she had just been shouted at in an unfriendly way. It is possible she might feel more relaxed in the mental health unit. Further medical treatment will depend on test results.
5. Joanne appeared to differ from the others because she put herself in Katia's place and tried to see things from her point of view as someone who is confused, frightened and frustrated.

Further reading

Griffith, R and Tengnah, C (2017) *Law and professional issues in nursing* (4th edn). London: Sage/Learning Matters.

Helpful guide linking ethical principles with law and applying them to nursing practice.

Melia, K (2013) *Ethics for nursing and healthcare practice.* London: Sage.

Informative account of ethical and moral theories and principles applied to nursing and healthcare.

Useful websites

www.healthwatch.co.uk/rights

Website of the consumer rights watchdog for healthcare listing eight patient rights including 'A safe and dignified quality service' and 'To be listened to' that nurses and other healthcare workers need to address.

www.humanrightsinhealthcare.nhs.uk

Human rights in healthcare website. Click 'Good practice' to look in detail at case studies such as Mersey Care learning disability service or click 'Advice & support' to download a service users' 'FREDA' booklet.

www.nmc.org.uk

NMC website explaining its role in setting professional and educational standards, regulating nursing and midwifery practice and investigating concerns about nurses or midwives, plus access to NMC publications.

www.nursingtimes.net

Very informative website packed with wide-ranging topical, ethical issues challenging nurses.

www.rcn.org.uk

Royal College of Nursing website where you can find and download useful resources concerning all eight of the RCN principles of nursing practice including a reference card, a poster and a workbook.

Chapter 10
Accountability for nursing decisions

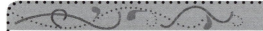

NMC Standards for Pre-registration Nursing Education

This chapter will address the following competencies:

Domain 1: Professional values

1. All nurses must practise with confidence according to *The Code: professional standards of practice and behaviour for nurses and midwives* (NMC, 2015), and within other recognised ethical and legal frameworks. They must be able to recognise and address ethical challenges relating to people's choices and decision-making about their care, and act within the law to help them and their families and carers find acceptable solutions.

Domain 3: Nursing practice and decision-making

6. All nurses must practise safely by being aware of the correct use, limitations and hazards of common interventions, including nursing activities, treatments, and the use of medical devices and equipment. The nurse must be able to evaluate their use, report any concerns promptly through appropriate channels and modify care where necessary to maintain safety. They must contribute to the collection of local and national data and formulation of policy on risks, hazards and adverse outcomes.

NMC Essential Skills Clusters

This chapter will address the following ESCs:

Cluster: Organisational aspects of care

11. People can trust the newly registered graduate nurse to safeguard children and adults from vulnerable situations and support and protect them from harm.

16. People can trust the newly registered graduate nurse to safely lead, co-ordinate and manage care.

20. People can trust the newly registered graduate nurse to select and manage medical devices safely.

Chapter aims

By the end of this chapter, you should be able to:

- explain what accountability for nursing decisions means;
- identify different parties to whom nurses are accountable;
- understand ways in which accountability is applied in practice;
- discuss protective, deterrent, regulatory and educative functions;
- appreciate why nurses are accountable for their decisions, actions or omissions.

Introduction

This chapter explores accountability for nursing decisions. We are held to account for what we do as nurses, at all times, and this includes meeting standards set out in the nursing and midwifery *Code*:

> *The Code contains the professional standards that registered nurses and midwives must uphold. UK nurses and midwives must act in line with The Code … While you can interpret the values and principles set out in The Code in a range of different practice settings, they are not negotiable or discretionary. We can take action if registered nurses or midwives fail to uphold The Code. In serious cases, this can include removing them from the register.*
> (NMC, 2015, p2)

In the case study a ward manager challenges a student nurse about his behaviour.

Case study: Whistling in the treatment room

Reggie is a first-year student on an adult nursing programme. While on placement in a medical ward he is shown how to dispose of used needles and syringes properly. Reggie has a habit of whistling tunes quite loudly when he is not working directly with the patients on the ward. One day, after giving an injection to a patient (under the supervision of his mentor) he is directed to dispose of the used needle and syringe in the treatment room. True to form, he starts whistling a tune rather loudly while alone in the treatment room. The ward manager can hear him while she is talking to a relative at the other end of the ward. She excuses herself for a moment to ask a staff nurse to go and tell Reggie to stop whistling.

The case study shows how everything we do as nurses is open to scrutiny or criticism by others and may incur sanctions if our behaviour is deemed to be inappropriate. Activity 10.1 asks you to think about the case study a bit more as a way of beginning to explore nurses' accountability.

Activity 10.1   *Leadership and management*

In this activity you are asked to explore how nurses should *be aware at all times of how [their] behaviour can affect and influence the behaviour of other people* (NMC, 2015, p15) and to reflect on what Reggie and the ward manager did by answering the following questions.

1.   Do you think Reggie was justified in whistling? If so, why?
2.   Do you think the ward manager was justified in stopping him from whistling? If so, why?

Some possible answers can be found at the end of the chapter.

Activity 10.1 illustrates a key feature of accountability: the need to justify decisions and actions we take as nurses (even seemingly innocuous activities such as whistling in the treatment room) because everything we do impacts upon patient care and the reputation of the profession. This chapter explores what accountability for nursing decisions means, who we are accountable to, how we are held to account and why being accountable is so important in decision-making. In doing so we will understand:

*   how nurses' accountability fits into the bigger picture of NHS accountability;
*   how it is applied alongside each of the perceptions of decision-making discussed in the other chapters;
*   the NMC's role regarding professional accountability;
*   how conceptions of nursing can be integrated and applied alongside accountability for nurses' clinical decision-making.

What is accountability?

Accountability for nursing decisions requires us, at all times, to be able to give an account of what we have done, what we are doing or what we intend doing, to those to whom we are accountable. It involves describing or explaining decisions and resulting actions, justifying why they are or were necessary and logically defending our decision-making processes and their outcomes when challenged to do so.

Accountability is a 'close cousin' of responsibility, with the latter associated with our particular roles as nurses and the various clinical activities we are expected to undertake. Nurses have always had many responsibilities in caring for patients, but it is only relatively recently that our professional autonomy has developed to a point where we are fully accountable for what we do. It requires a higher standard of education, which is why nursing has evolved into a graduate entry profession. Accountability is also linked to the development of evidence-based nursing practice because our decision-making and actions are more likely to be safe, effective and justifiable where they are supported by relevant research findings and principles of good practice. In the previous case study, the ward manager decided that Reggie's whistling was not justifiable. In the following case study a newly qualified nurse explains her understanding of accountability.

Case study: Being responsible for nursing decisions

Susan is in her first job as a staff nurse at a general hospital. In reflecting on the difference between being a student or a registered nurse she reveals her understanding of accountability.

'I've had to learn to think on my feet and make decisions on the spot. I need to be responsible and accountable for why I made those decisions. If someone asks why you are doing a certain procedure – like fitting anti-embolism stockings for a patient on bed rest to prevent the increased risk of deep vein thrombosis and pulmonary embolism – you need to be able to explain it is evidence-based and it works. You cannot just say, "because I'm the staff nurse!"'

The case study illustrates how accountability means knowing how what you propose to do is of benefit to patients, and being able to explain it to them so that they understand and consent to it. In Activity 10.2 you are asked to think about your own examples in this respect.

Activity 10.2   *Communication*

Think about your current or recent practice placements, and select three different examples of how you contributed to patient care. Did you do so because a colleague asked for help? Were you instructed to? Or did a patient ask for your help? Describe what you did for each patient by answering these questions.

- What were you doing for this patient?
- How do you know whether the patient consented to you doing this?
- Which health needs were your actions intended to address?
- How did you know that you were competent to perform these procedures?
- What knowledge, skills and attitudes did you apply in caring for this patient?

Now imagine that your link lecturer from the university asks you to evaluate the care you gave and answer these questions.

- How do you know whether you performed procedures at the required standard?
- How successful or unsuccessful were the outcomes of your interventions?
- What benefit did the patient experience and how can you be sure of this?
- What, if anything, would you do differently next time and why?

Write down your answers to each question. Discuss questions and responses with a colleague, and take turns to question and explain to each other the rationale for decisions and related actions. It will give you practice in explaining and defending your actions to others, which is at the heart of accountability for nursing decisions.

As this is for your own reflection, no outline answer is included for this activity.

Activity 10.2 helps clarify what accountability for nursing decisions means using questions we need to ask ourselves when caring for patients. Of course, nurses do not care for patients in isolation from other healthcare professionals, most of whom are also employed by the NHS. The NHS is accountable for the organisation, management and delivery of a high standard of healthcare throughout the country, and our professional accountability as nurses therefore complements the goals of the NHS. Following an extensive review (DH, 2008a), principles and values were described in 2009 of an NHS Constitution that all personnel (doctors, nurses, allied health professions, support services, managers) have to abide by. The Constitution also identifies the responsibilities of service users in positively contributing to their own care. Table 10.1 summarises key principles and values of the 2013 edition of the NHS Constitution.

The values identified in Table 10.1 complement those of nurses and other health professionals, and it is good to see that these are used to inform the principles of organising health services.

NHS principles	NHS values
1. The NHS provides a comprehensive service available to all.	• Everyone counts (healthcare for all, no one is left out and all have a part to play in promoting and achieving personal and community health).
2. Access to NHS services is based on clinical need not an individual's ability to pay.	
3. The NHS aspires to highest standards of excellence and professionalism.	• Compassion (comfort and relieve suffering through being caring, kind and attentive).
4. The NHS aspires to put patients at the heart of everything it does/services must reflect the needs and preferences of patients, their families and their carers.	• Respect and dignity (value each person as individual with own priorities, abilities, needs).
5. The NHS works across organisational boundaries and in partnerships with other organisations in the interest of patients, local communities and the wider population.	• Working together for patients (put needs of patients and communities first and overcome any restrictions of organisational boundaries/speak up when things go wrong).
6. The NHS is committed to providing best value for taxpayers' money and the most effective, fair and sustainable use of finite resources.	• Improving lives (strive to improve health and wellbeing and people's experiences of NHS).
7. The NHS is accountable to the public, communities and patients that it serves.	• Commitment to quality of care (earn trust by high standards of care – welcome feedback to learn from mistakes and build on successes).

Table 10.1: The NHS Constitution

Source: Adapted from DH, 2013a

They also reinforce the importance of creating and maintaining a culture of compassionate care in the NHS (DH, 2012a). The creation of the NHS Constitution was influenced by some well-publicised instances of appalling healthcare associated with poor management. These included being unresponsive to local needs while pursuing national health targets, inadequate leadership regarding infection control and lack of suitably qualified staff, facilities and equipment to cope with high clinical demands. Nurses and other health professionals are always personally accountable for the quality of care that they give, but if they are understaffed, under-resourced, poorly supervised and overworked, it is more difficult to maintain high standards.

In order to rectify this, the Francis Report (2013) – a public inquiry into serious failings at Mid Staffordshire NHS Foundation Trust – recommended a *patients first culture* and a *duty of candour* (honesty/openness/transparency) by all organisations and individuals providing healthcare. This includes publishing all complaints about patient care on hospital websites, encouraging staff to speak up if something is wrong and banning 'gagging clauses' used by employers to stop staff revealing their concerns in public. The NHS Constitution was updated in 2013 in response to these recommendations (e.g. *speak up when things go wrong*). Recognising that patient needs and professional values should have more influence in structuring and managing services is vital in making NHS services more accountable to the needs of local communities. As nurses, we are accountable for upholding both our professional standards and principles, and values of the NHS Constitution.

Who are we accountable to?

First and foremost we are accountable to the patients, clients or service users to whom we owe a duty of care. We are accountable to the wider public, who indirectly pay for what we do via tax and national insurance. We are accountable to employers (e.g. the NHS), who enable our contact with patients by assigning us duties in employment contracts and job descriptions. Nurses are professionally accountable to the NMC to *put the interests of people using or needing our services first* (NMC, 2015, p4). Like other citizens, we are accountable to society in abiding by civil law (e.g. Human Rights Act 1998: see Chapter 9) and criminal law (e.g. Theft Act 1968). Nursing students are also accountable to universities for their academic progress, and to clinical mentors or assessors who act as 'gatekeepers' to the profession in judging their professional suitability. Having clarified what accountability is and who we are accountable to, we can define accountability as follows:

> *Accountability in decision-making is being answerable to patients, public, employers, NMC and the law for the consequences of actions, and having to explain, justify and defend our decisions.*

How do we demonstrate accountability?

In this section we will explore how we demonstrate accountability for nursing decisions through observation of our practice, record keeping and all types and instances of our decision-making.

Accountability and observation of our practice

Just as we use observation skills in assessing those in our care, we ourselves are continually observed by service users and members of the healthcare team. When we are attentive and responsive to patients' needs and preferences, we are demonstrating our accountability to them and they are more likely to feel well cared for and to evaluate the experience positively. If a patient is unhappy about the way we are caring for them, they are at liberty to make a complaint. We are then obliged to listen, apologise for any upset caused and take action to remedy concerns. Sometimes healthcare colleagues act as advocates on behalf of patients (like the ward manager in the earlier case study) if they judge a team member's behaviour needs adjusting in patients' best interests. It is not always possible to have a team around you to observe, support and supervise what you are doing, for example, if you are nursing in community settings. Such nurses therefore need to be highly proficient. If they are not, patients can suffer, as the following case study describes.

Case study: Switching off the life support by mistake

Jamie had a car accident in 2002 that left him paralysed from the neck down (tetraplegic). It means he cannot breathe unless a machine (ventilator) is connected to his windpipe via a hole in his neck (tracheostomy). In spite of his high level of disability, Jamie was cared for at home. He was mentally alert, able to engage in meaningful discussions, used voice-activated computer technology to access the internet and write emails and got about in a motorised wheelchair (if helped to get in and out). Jamie's main nursing need concerned his breathing as he was totally dependent on his ventilator machine. The NHS Trust entrusted his care to a private nursing agency. Jamie became worried about the quality of care he received and had a camera installed in January 2009 to video his care. It was done quite openly and there was a sign to inform nurses the camera was recording so that Jamie's family could check that he was all right.

Soon after the camera was installed, an agency nurse who had had no training or experience in the use of ventilator machines was attending to Jamie. The nurse found a switch that was turned on and decided to turn it off; an alarm sounded (warning not to turn the ventilator machine off). Jamie could not speak without air so he frantically made a clicking noise with his tongue on the roof of his mouth (as he had been trained to do in an emergency) to show he was in distress. The nurse attempted to resuscitate him but wrongly placed a portable ventilation bag (Ambu bag) over his mouth instead of the opening in his neck (the only way air could get to his lungs). Someone dialled 999, paramedics arrived, resuscitated Jamie and turned the ventilator machine back on. Jamie survived but suffered serious brain damage due to 20 minutes without oxygen. These events were captured by Jamie's camera, recorded onto his computer and found by his sister. The nurse was suspended subject to an NMC investigation, and the NHS Trust instigated a review of policies with a view to preventing such tragedies from happening again in future.
(Adapted from BBC, 2010)

Jamie's case study begs many questions about the organisation and delivery of care in the community, such as: Why did the NHS Trust not have their own trained district nurses to oversee such specialist care? Why did the nursing agency delegate Jamie's care to a nurse who was not qualified to carry it out? Here we will focus on the nurse's own accountability for her decision-making and actions, as revealed by the video evidence.

No criminal charges were brought against the nurse, which means the police believed it was accidental rather than a deliberate attempt to harm Jamie. There was no justification for switching off the ventilator machine. Following an investigation and formal hearing, the nurse in this case was struck off the NMC register in 2012 due to impairment of practice that posed an unacceptable risk to the public.

Without Jamie's foresight in fitting a camera we would not have evidence of what happened. It highlights the point that we demonstrate our accountability for providing safe, competent nursing care each moment we are on duty. It is unusual for this to be observed and video recorded, but in a sense we need to imagine that this is happening all the time. If we stop to think, 'Would I be happy for a video of how I just spoke to a patient or gave an injection to be seen by the NMC?' it would remind us not to do anything that we cannot justify being in the best interests of patients. In Activity 10.3 you are asked to explore various implications of the case study in more detail.

Activity 10.3   *Critical thinking*

The case study shows what can go wrong when nurses find themselves out of their depth and carry out tasks they are not competent to perform using medical devices unfamiliar to them. In this activity you are asked to reflect on how the nurse in the case study might have avoided endangering Jamie's life, permanently injuring him and increasing his already severe disability. You are then asked to relate this to your own practice. Please answer the following questions.

1. When the agency nurse discovered the severity of Jamie's disability and realised she did not have the knowledge or skills to care for him competently, what should she have done?
2. What may have stopped her from acknowledging she lacked competence to care for Jamie?
3. When the agency nurse noticed that a switch had been left on and was concerned about it, what alternative action should she have taken rather than turning it off?
4. What may have stopped her from deciding to take more appropriate alternative action?
5. If you were to be asked to perform a procedure you do not feel competent in, what would you do?
6. If you find a switch on an unfamiliar medical device left switched on, what would you do?

Some possible answers can be found at the end of the chapter.

Activity 10.3 and Jamie's case study underline how important it is for nurses to know what they are doing, and not do what they are not competent to perform. In order to be accountable we have to justify our decision-making. We can only justify decision-making if we understand how our actions are of benefit to patients, including reference to relevant supporting evidence. We may also be able to justify a decision not to perform a procedure where we can argue we lack the skills to do so safely and effectively. This would not excuse us from ensuring the patient is attended to by someone who has the required level of clinical competence. So far we have looked at how observations of our practice can be used in holding us to account for decision-making. We will now look at how written records of care can also be used for this purpose.

Accountability and written records of our practice

Just as we need to base decision-making and nursing activities on relevant research evidence, current policies and clinical guidelines, we are also required to keep up-to-date written records as evidence of the care we have given. The importance of good record keeping is spelled out in *The Code* (NMC, 2015, p9), as follows:

> **10 Keep clear and accurate records relevant to your practice** *(This includes but is not limited to patient records. It includes all records that are relevant to your scope of practice). To achieve this you must:*
>
> *10.1 complete all records at the time or as soon possible after an event, recording if the notes are written sometime after the event*
>
> *10.2 identify any risks or problems that have arisen and the steps taken to deal with them, so that colleagues who use the records have all the information they need*
>
> *10.3 complete all records accurately and without falsification, taking immediate and appropriate action if you become aware that someone has not kept to these requirements*
>
> *10.4 attribute any entries you make in any paper or electronic records to yourself, making sure they are clearly written, dated and timed, and do not include unnecessary abbreviations, jargon or speculation*
>
> *10.5 take all steps to make sure that all records are kept securely, and*
>
> *10.6 collect, treat and store all data and research findings appropriately.*

Handwritten or electronic notes, reflective journals, observation charts, drug charts, care plans and assessment forms contribute to an audit trail of decision-making that we can be asked to explain, justify and defend. In the next case study a newly qualified nurse shows how problems can occur when record keeping is inaccurate or not kept up to date in administering medicines.

Case study: Signing the drug chart

Tracy registered as a nurse six months ago and has recently completed additional training in administering intravenous fluids and medication. Robert is due to receive a powerful intravenous antibiotic, and Tracy checks the drug with another nurse before attending to him. After giving the antibiotic Robert's bedside telephone rings and he asks Tracy if she'd mind telling whoever it is that he is having treatment and not 'up to talking' at the moment. Tracy obliges, puts the phone down and leaves Robert

continued . . .

to rest, completely forgetting to sign that he had the antibiotic on the drug chart. When the next shift takes over they give Robert an extra dose because there is no record of him having had the antibiotic earlier. When the mistake is discovered a clinical incident form is filled in. Matron asks Tracy to apologise to Robert and to inform his consultant about it, which she does. She feels terribly embarrassed and vows not to be so easily distracted from finishing what she is doing, and to make sure she remembers to sign the drug chart in future. Robert did not suffer any ill effects, but Tracy felt it was more by luck than judgement on her part.

The case study highlights how important accurate record keeping is in documenting patient care and the potential problems of not doing so. It also reinforces the point that nurses are not only accountable for what they do but also for what they do not do (not signing drug chart).

If Robert's bedside phone had not rung, then Tracy would not have been distracted from signing the chart. As nurses we cannot simply hope that nothing distracts us from carrying out procedures. There will always be 'a phone call' or some other distraction, so we have to find better ways of dealing with them. Activity 10.4 asks you to explore Tracy's accountability for her decision-making.

Activity 10.4   *Decision-making*

Decision-making involves selecting a course of action from the available alternatives. In this activity you are asked to evaluate Tracy's decision-making, and to consider what else she might have done and what can be learnt from such mistakes. Please answer the following questions.

1. Do you think Tracy was justified in not signing the drug chart? If yes, why? If not, why not?
2. Do you think Tracy was justified in answering the phone? If yes, why? If not, why not?
3. What alternative options were available to Tracy when Robert's bedside phone rang?
4. Do you think the matron was justified in asking Tracy to apologise to Robert and inform the consultant about the mistake that had been made? If yes, why? If not, why not?
5. Look at the NMC requirements of good record keeping (above) and select three that were not met by Tracy. How would signing a drug chart address these points?
6. Given that Robert did not appear to suffer any ill effects from Tracy's oversight, why do you think it is important that she learns not to make the same mistake again?

Some possible answers can be found at the end of the chapter.

The case study highlights a 'fine line' between nurses helping patients (beneficence) and not harming patients (non-maleficence). Tracy's caring instinct was to do what Robert wanted by answering the phone but this incident taught her to think more carefully about doing so. By allowing herself to be distracted from completing the intravenous procedure properly, rather than helping Robert, she exposed him to possible danger. In being held to account for her mistake Tracy was made acutely aware that being a caring person is not enough to be an effective nurse. We also need to be vigilant in continually assessing risks associated with our decision-making and related actions, and then control such risks to avoid endangering patients. This is easier said than done, but it is vital that we do so.

As the healthcare professionals having most contact with patients, nurses have more decision-making opportunities in assessing and addressing their needs and preferences than others. We are accountable for a great many nursing decisions every day. It is why observations of our practice by patients and others, and written records of what we have done, are key sources of evidence in holding us to account for our decision-making. Through clinical governance this is happening all the time at a local level, as shown in the case study. Tracy was held to account for confusing kindness with her duty of care to competently complete the intravenous procedure and sign the drug chart. By deviating from standardised procedure (Chapter 5) Tracy exposed Robert to greater risk and left herself open to criticism.

It is fortunate the outcome of her mistake did not adversely affect Robert's health and well-being. Knowing that the outcome could have been worse emphasises the importance of learning from and avoiding such mistakes in future. Being accountable goes hand in hand with striving to improve the care we give to patients. We saw in Jamie's case study that nurses are required to account for decision-making at a national level if the outcomes of mistakes are more serious. This leads us to look at how the NMC *Code* reminds us of our accountability in all aspects of decision-making.

Accountability in all aspects of decision-making

Accountability has been identified in this book as a decision-making theme in its own right because knowing that we are answerable for our decisions as nurses affects how we make them. However, in itself accountability does not tell us how to make a decision – only that it should be justifiable as being in the best interests of patients. In practice, each perception of decision-making discussed in this book needs to be combined with accountability because without it there is no way of confirming that we fulfilled our duty of care to patients.

Table 10.2 shows how to apply relevant extracts from *The Code* (NMC, 2015) regarding our professional accountability as nurses alongside the other perceptions of decision-making. In Robert's case study there is a clash between collaborative and standardised decision-making as Tracy interrupted the intravenous procedure to answer Robert's phone for him. If we apply Table 10.2 to Jamie's case study, the nurse did not demonstrate her accountability in recognising and working within the limits of her competence (reflective), and informing her employers to send a suitably qualified and experienced nurse to care for Jamie (experience and intuition).

It may seem ironic that as nurses aspire to more professional autonomy they encounter more accountability for their decision-making and nursing interventions. This is an in-built safeguard to protect patients as the power of nurses and other health professionals to make vital

Perceptions of decision-making	Extracts from NMC *Code* (2015) linking perceptions of decision-making to professional accountability
Collaborative	Work in partnership with people to make sure you deliver care effectively (p4); Respect the level to which people receiving care want to be involved in decisions about their own health, wellbeing and care; Act in partnership with those receiving care, helping to access relevant health and social care, information and support when they need it (p5); Communicate clearly; Use terms that people in your care, colleagues and the public can understand (p7); Work co-operatively; Respect the skills, expertise and contributions of your colleagues, referring matters to them when appropriate; Provide honest, accurate and constructive feedback to colleagues (p8); Deal with differences of opinion with colleagues by discussion and informed debate, respecting their views and opinions and behaving in a professional way at all times (p9); Be accountable for your decisions to delegate tasks and duties to other people (p10); Make a timely and appropriate referral to another practitioner when it is in the best interests of the individual needing any action, treatment or care (p11).
Observation	Recognise when people are anxious or in distress and respond compassionately and politely; Pay special attention to promoting wellbeing, preventing ill health and meeting the changing health and care needs of people during all life stages (p5); Complete all records at the time or as soon after an event, recording if the notes are written sometime after the event; Identify any risks or problems that have arisen and the steps taken to deal with them, so that colleagues who use the records have all the information they need (p9); Accurately assess signs of normal or worsening physical and mental health in the person receiving care (p11).
Systematic	Make sure that people's physical, social and psychological needs are assessed and responded to (5); Work with colleagues to evaluate the quality of your work and that of the team (p8); Keep clear and accurate records relevant to your practice (p9); Make sure that the care or treatment you advise on, prescribe, supply, dispense or administer for each person is compatible with any other care or treatment they are receiving, including (where possible) over-the-counter medicines (p14); Stay objective and have clear professional boundaries at all times with people in your care (p15).
Standardised	Always practise in line with the best available evidence (p7); Keep to appropriate guidelines when giving advice on using controlled drugs and recording the prescribing, supply, dispensing or administration of controlled drugs; Take account of current evidence, knowledge and

(Continued)

Perceptions of decision-making	Extracts from NMC *Code* (2015) linking perceptions of decision-making to professional accountability
	developments in reducing mistakes and the effect of them and the impact of human factors and system failures; Keep to and promote recommended practice in relation to controlling and preventing infection (p14); Keep to and uphold the standards and values set out in the *Code*; Keep to the laws of the country in which you are practising (p15).
Prioritising	Act without delay if you believe that there is a risk to patient safety or public protection; Raise and, if necessary, escalate any concerns you may have about patient safety, or the level of care people are receiving in your workplace or any other healthcare setting (p12); Acknowledge and act on all concerns raised to you, investigating escalating or dealing with those concerns where it is appropriate for you to do so (p13); Be aware of, and reduce as far as possible, any potential for harm associated with your practice (p14); Identify priorities, manage time, staff and resources effectively and deal with risk to make sure that the quality of care or service you deliver is maintained and improved, putting the needs of those receiving care or services first (p18).
Experience and intuition	Share your knowledge and experience for the benefit of people receiving care and your colleagues (p8); Only delegate tasks and duties that are within the other person's scope of competence, making sure that they fully understand your instructions (p10); Ask for help from a suitably qualified and experienced healthcare professional to carry out any action or procedure that is beyond the limits of your competence (p11); Only act in an emergency within the limits of your knowledge and competence (p12).
Reflective	Maintain the knowledge and skills you need for safe and effective practice (p7); Gather and reflect on feedback from a variety of sources, using it to improve your practice and performance (p9); Recognise and work within the limits of your competence (p11); Use all complaints as a form of feedback and an opportunity for reflection and learning to improve practice (p18).
Ethical sensitivity	Treat people as individuals and uphold their dignity; Respect and uphold people's human rights (p4); Respect, support and document a person's right to accept or refuse care and treatment; Act as an advocate for the vulnerable, challenging poor practice and discriminatory attitudes and behaviour relating to their care; Act in the best interests of people at all times (p5); Make sure that you get properly informed consent and

	document it before carrying out any action; Respect people's right to privacy and confidentiality (p6); Be open and candid with all service users about all aspects of care and treatment, including when any mistakes or harm have taken place (p11); Act with honesty and integrity at all times, treating people fairly and without discrimination, bullying or harassment (p15).
Confidence	Support students' and colleagues' learning to help them develop their professional competence and confidence (p9); Promote professionalism and trust. You should display a personal commitment to the standards of practice and behaviour set out in *The Code*. You should be a model of integrity and leadership for others to aspire to. This should lead to trust and confidence in the profession from patients, people receiving care, other healthcare professionals and the public (p15).

Table 10.2: Nurses' professional accountability in relation to perceptions of decision-making

decisions regarding people's lives is tempered by the requirement that such decisions be open to scrutiny by others. This leads us on to clarifying why it is that accountability for nursing decisions is so important.

Why is accountability important?

So far we have established that accountability means having to account for (explain and justify) our decisions to patients, public, employers and the nursing profession, who observe our practice and may scrutinise written records of the care we have provided. At this point we need to be clear about the purpose of professional accountability in nursing. According to Griffith and Tengnah (2017), accountability has four functions – *protective, deterrent, regulatory* and *educative*. We will now explore what this means by relating these four functions of accountability to nursing decisions.

Protective function

This is the primary aim of professional accountability for nursing decisions. Our first duty as nurses is not to harm patients (non-maleficence) by our actions or lack of action (Chapter 9). Potential benefits of patient care can be undermined by unprofessional behaviour and by errors. The NMC is responsible for protecting the public by investigating complaints about nurses' fitness to practise and, if necessary, instigating sanctions. Sanctions include: (i) a caution not to repeat behaviour; (ii) making a condition of practice (e.g. requiring nurse to have more training or supervision in order to continue practising); (iii) suspension for up to one year (case reviewed at the end of suspension period); and (iv) a striking off order (nurse removed from NMC register).

In 2015–2016, the NMC received 5415 new referrals concerning allegations about nurses' and midwives' fitness to practise. This represents 0.8 per cent of the total number of registered nurses and midwives, 692,550 as at 31 March 2016 (NMC, 2016). The referrals were made by employers (41 per cent), patients/service users/public (25 per cent), self-referral (10 per cent), NMC registrar (6 per cent), other regulators (3 per cent), police (3 per cent) and various other sources. The allegations before the NMC range from lack of competence to serious professional misconduct.

Between April 2015 and March 2016 the NMC instigated 809 sanctions against nurses and midwives (i.e. 15 per cent of 5,415 referrals), including 261 striking off orders. The next case study provides examples of real cases where nurses have been struck off the NMC register.

Case study: Striking off orders for professional misconduct

These are examples from all four pathways of nurses who received striking off orders from the NMC register when charges of professional misconduct and impairment of their fitness to practise were judged to be proven.

- *A practice nurse (adult pathway) was dishonest in falsely claiming to hold three post-registration specialist qualifications in securing employment and in gaining further promotion. The nurse also breached a patient's confidentiality.*
- *A mental health nurse engaged in an inappropriate sexual relationship with a patient in an acute mental health unit he was working in and also after the patient's discharge, and failed to report professional boundary issues with supervisors or managers.*
- *A learning disabilities nurse at a special school for children with learning disabilities failed to carry out a physical assessment on a highly vulnerable, distressed child (who had fractured an ankle) and failed to refer the child for a medical assessment, dismissing the child as wanting 'molly coddling'. The nurse also falsified records of supervision meetings with a junior nurse.*
- *A child pathway nurse was convicted of 11 counts of downloading indecent images of children, including depictions of adults abusing children. The nurse was sentenced to 12 months' imprisonment, ordered to sign the Sex Offenders Register and placed on an indefinite Sexual Offences Prevention Order.*

The case study shows that where nurses' decisions and actions are unjustifiable and indefensible, the NMC has a duty to protect the public by making nurses accountable for their actions, including preventing them from continuing to practise. This is echoed in a letter from Robert Francis QC to the Secretary of State for Health that accompanied the Francis Report (2013); it reads as follows.

> *Make all those who provide care for patients – individuals and organisations – properly accountable for what they do to ensure that the public is protected from those not fit to provide such a service.*

This may seem small comfort for patients who have suffered from poor care or abuse. They or their families may be entitled to claim compensation from NHS Trusts and nurses in recognition that their health and wellbeing have not been protected due to negligent care and indefensible decision-making.

Deterrent function

The best type of protection is to prevent mistakes in healthcare from occurring in the first place. The knowledge that we are always being observed, our performance evaluated and records of decision-making and care delivery audited, reminds us always to act professionally. Hearing about nurses being suspended or dismissed from their jobs, or found unfit to practise and struck off the NMC register, underlines how we are accountable to a higher authority that has the power to take away our livelihood. This discourages us from emulating unprofessional behaviour that undermines the public's trust and confidence in nurses. For example, one of the nurses involved in administering a fatal amount of sodium chloride to a young baby (Chapter 9) was not only investigated by the NMC regarding her role in this but she was also sacked by the NHS Trust for gross misconduct. She had uploaded onto her social networking site photos of herself asleep next to (and supposedly looking after) the baby who later died. Imagine how the parents of the baby boy would have felt about this. By sacking the nurse, her employers clearly showed that such behaviour is unacceptable and will not be tolerated. It is a 'wake-up call' for other nurses to keep their professional and personal lives separate in relation to social networking sites. Standards of practice and behaviour in *The Code* (NMC, 2015, p16) emphasise this point:

> *20.10 Use all forms of spoken, written and digital communication (including social media and networking sites) responsibly, respecting the right to privacy of others at all times.*

The deterrent function of accountability therefore gives us professional boundaries that it is foolish to cross.

Regulatory function

Whereas the deterrent function dissuades us from doing what we should not do, the regulatory function of accountability tells us what we should do to justify public trust in nurses. *The Code* for nurses and midwives lists the professional standards of practice and behaviour that we need to demonstrate in this respect (NMC, 2015). This is the regulatory framework defining what we do as nurses, and by complying with it we demonstrate our professional accountability. If we adhere to *The Code* in our clinical practice, we increase the chances that our decision-making and nursing actions will benefit rather than harm patients (as outlined in Table 10.2, pages 177–9). Complying with *The Code* does not guarantee that complications will not occur, but if they do, we are able to show that we did what we could to achieve the best possible outcome for patients. In this way abiding by *The Code* not only protects patients, it also protects our reputation as nurses.

Other regulatory frameworks we have to abide by include the NHS Constitution specifying principles and values all parties need to respect throughout the NHS. NICE or other evidence-based clinical guidelines, underpinning standardised decision-making (Chapter 5), provide a practical

Relevant Act or Order	Examples of application in nursing
Health Care and Associated Professions (Indemnity Arrangements) Order 2014	'Have in place an indemnity arrangement which provides appropriate cover for any practice you take on as a nurse or midwife in the United Kingdom' (NMC, 2015, p11).
Health and Social Care Act 2012	Nursing representation on clinical commissioning groups of local healthcare services.
Equality Act 2010	No discrimination regarding age, sex, race or disability.
Health Act 2009	Apply principles and values of the NHS Constitution.
Health and Social Care Act 2008	Co-operate with Care Quality Commission inquiries.
Mental Health Act 1983/2007	Voluntary or compulsory criteria to treat mental disorder.
Mental Capacity Act 2005	Safeguarding rights of vulnerable people if unable to make decisions for themselves.
Nursing and Midwifery Order 2001	Comply with NMC code of professional, ethical conduct.
Freedom of Information Act 2000	Patients' right of access to view records of their care.
Data Protection Act 1998	Only authorised access to patients' confidential data.
Human Rights Act 1998	Respect patients' right to life and to dignified treatment.
Children Act 1989	Duty to report suspected non-accidental injury of a child.
Health and Safety at Work Act 1974	Obligation to report safety concerns within clinical areas.
Misuse of Drugs Act 1971	Safely store, record, give (if prescribed) controlled drugs.

Table 10.3: Examples of legally enforceable regulatory frameworks

regulatory framework for everyday use. Many regulatory frameworks influencing our clinical practice have a legal basis – see Table 10.3.

Table 10.3 gives an indication of many legally enforceable regulatory frameworks that impact on our role and duty as nurses. It may seem a lot for us to take in, but in practice many of the policies and procedures in clinical areas incorporate relevant aspects of this myriad of legislation. For example, whilst it is your duty to *make sure that you have an appropriate indemnity arrangement in place* (NMC, 2015, p11), which enables patients to seek justice and claim compensation for any clinical negligence, in most NHS settings this is covered by the employer's 'duty of care' to patients and their 'vicarious liability' for employees' actions. If you are an RCN/other professional association member, personal indemnity insurance is also usually included in the membership fee. This may be of help if you are not be covered by the 'vicarious liability' rule, for example, if you are self-employed. In addition, membership of a professional association usually entitles you to support and advice, and possibly legal representation, if any allegations are made against you. The more we delve into accountability, the more there is to learn, and we will look into this a bit more now.

Educative function

Accountability requires us to explain, justify and defend our actions to others, and we cannot do this unless we think about and articulate reasons and evidence supporting our decision-making. Hence, the very act of demonstrating our accountability is potentially educational, prompting us to be aware of what we are doing and why, risks associated with our actions, how competent we feel in managing these and whether we have given anyone cause to make a complaint. Simon, a newly qualified nurse, identified three questions to sum up his understanding of accountability: *What happens if it goes wrong? What happens to the patient? What happens to me?* In the next case study, Sean, another newly qualified nurse, described a situation he found quite challenging in deciding whether or not to give a patient prescribed discretionary medication.

Case study: PRN medication

Sean's first staff nurse job is in an acute mental health unit where Nick, aged 26, is being treated for anxiety and depression. Along with his regular medication Nick is prescribed an extra dose of anti-anxiety PRN medication. PRN is short for pro re nata (Latin), meaning to be taken when required. Sean had to use his discretion in judging whether it was appropriate to give the additional medication, given that it could be addictive and Nick had a history of drug abuse.

'I noticed Nick was making a habit of coming every day for the PRN medication and I wondered whether he really needed it, or was misusing it. It was almost as if he treated it as an additional regular supply but that was not what it was intended for. Many times I did not feel he looked particularly agitated to warrant the PRN dose. Then I thought he might feel agitated but not show visible signs, and the PRN was prescribed so maybe I should give it to him when he asks. I decided to ask Nick what he was agitated about, and a couple of times he just started smiling, so I didn't give him the PRN on those days. There were other days when he could give a valid reason why he was feeling stressed, and so I felt more confident giving it then. It was something I reviewed all the time to try to ensure the PRN medication was used for therapeutic reasons.'

The case study shows how Sean applied accountability in nursing decisions. He could have simply given the PRN medication every time Nick asked, but he felt this was unjustifiable when the evidence suggested additional medication was not required. Using Simon's questions as a guide, we can review Sean's decision-making.

- *What happens if it goes wrong?* If Sean got it wrong, he would either give the PRN medication when Nick did not really need it or not give it when he did.
- *What happens to the patient?* Nick would either be over- or under-medicated, neither of which would be therapeutic.
- *What happens to me?* Sean would either be colluding with drug misuse by Nick or upsetting Nick by not trusting him when he was genuinely in need of PRN anti-anxiety medication.

Conceptions of nursing	Accountability in decision-making
Caring	Ensuring PRN medication is beneficial and not harmful to Nick.
Listening and being there	Give Nick time to explain what might be worrying him.
Practical procedures	Safely giving or not giving PRN medication, as appropriate.
Knowledge and understanding	Anti-anxiety drugs, doses, side-effects, uses and abuses.
Communicating	Asking Nick directly what he is feeling agitated about.
Patience	Control possible sense of irritation that Nick is 'trying it on'.
Teamwork	Entrusted by doctor to decide if PRN medication is needed.
Paperwork and electronic record	Recording medication given, and the interactions with Nick.
Empathising and non-judgemental	Appreciate that Nick may genuinely need PRN medication.
Professional	Maintaining good relationship without colluding with Nick.

Table 10.4: Integrating conceptions of nursing and accountability in decision-making

There are many ways we can explain, justify and defend our actions, and Table 10.4 relates Sean's accountability for decision-making to conceptions of nursing.

Table 10.4 shows how accountability for nursing decisions might be explained with reference to the ten conceptions of nursing. Matching accountability to each of the conceptions of nursing requires reflective learning, which contributes to its educative function. In Activity 10.5 you are asked to apply this to your own practice placement experience.

Activity 10.5   *Reflection*

Although, as a student, you are not fully accountable for patient care, you are accountable for making good use of your learning opportunities in practice placements. With this in mind, identify an example when you were working with a patient and felt you made a meaningful contribution to their care. Then adapt Table 10.4 to map your example against the ten conceptions of nursing, indicating how justifiable your actions were in the same way that we did for Sean. It should help you to integrate an awareness of accountability with your development as a nurse.

As this activity is for your own private reflection, there is no outline answer included.

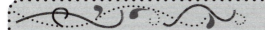

Chapter summary

This chapter discussed the nature of accountability for nursing decisions and how this requires us to be able to explain, justify and defend our decision-making. We noted that compliance with the NMC *Code* facilitates our professional accountability and that we also have to adhere to the principles and values of the NHS Constitution. We identified that we are primarily accountable to service users but also to employers, the NMC and the law for our decision-making, actions and mistakes. We looked at how we need to demonstrate accountability in everything we do as we are being constantly observed by patients, colleagues and others. Written records of the care we give also provide evidence of our decision-making, and whether it appears justified. We established that accountability is married to each of the other perceptions of decision-making discussed in this book, and this was supported with reference to the NMC's *Code*. We examined why accountability is so important in protecting patients and the wider public by ensuring that nurses deemed unfit for practice forfeit the right to do so. It was argued that this can help deter nurses from making the same mistakes. We also looked at how a range of legally enforceable frameworks – not just the NMC *Code* – regulate our decision-making and conduct.

It was argued that being continually aware of our accountability for decision-making is educational as it prompts us to question our practice and examine the strength of supporting evidence. The strengths of accountability in clinical decision-making include constantly reminding us of our responsibility to our patients to provide safe and effective, patient-centred, evidence-based, high quality nursing care. Being accountable for our decisions and actions also endorses our professional status as knowledgeable and skilled nurses who can be trusted to deliver high quality care. The weaknesses of accountability include the sad reality that many patients received poor care before the nurses, other health professionals or NHS managers concerned were called to account for their failings. Topical case studies and related activities highlighted the challenges faced by nurses, what happens if things go wrong and how to apply accountability in clinical decision-making to ensure patients receive the best possible care.

Activities: brief outline answers

Activity 10.1: Leadership and management (page 168)

You may have included the following points.

1. Reggie's possible justification for whistling: boost morale, de-stress, relax, convey happiness at work; was not in direct contact with patients during the activity; unaware he was causing a distraction or disturbance.
2. Ward manager's possible justification to stop Reggie whistling: distracting her while talking to relative; relative could also have been distracted; it might be viewed as unprofessional behaviour in an acute medical setting; it could possibly disturb patients who need to rest; Reggie may not hear if a patient or colleague needs assistance; disposal of used needles/syringes part of infection control to be taken seriously.

Activity 10.3: Critical thinking (page 173)

You may have included the following points.

1. Phone nursing agency, talk to the duty manager, explain she was not able to care for Jamie safely or effectively as his needs were beyond her experience and training, and ask for a suitable replacement; explain to Jamie reason for the delay in attending to his care needs; request further training and supervision from agency before being asked to care for Jamie.
2. Fear that she might lose her job with nursing agency; too proud to admit ignorance; lack of critical awareness of risks posed to Jamie in attempting to care for him when she did not understand what she was doing; unfamiliarity with professional *Code* in nursing – *Recognise and work within the limits of your competence* (NMC, 2015, p11).
3. Leave the switch alone as she did not know what it was for and at that time Jamie was not in any distress so there was no reason to think leaving it switched on would harm him; up until the time the nurse turned off ventilator machine Jamie could speak, so if she was unsure about anything, she could have asked him, and he would have explained things to her.
4. She may have felt a compulsion 'to be seen to be doing something', not realising she was putting Jamie in grave danger. She may have underestimated Jamie's lucid mind (due to his physical disability) and not realised he was an expert in his own care who could advise her. Perhaps she didn't like being videoed and thought she was turning the camera off.
5. Admit you have not done it before or not reached a competent standard; request you observe a competent nurse performing the procedure before you attempt it; read up on the procedure – its purpose, equipment needed and technique; familiarise yourself with the patient concerned and how the procedure is intended to be of benefit regarding their medical condition; only then agree to perform the procedure under the watchful eye of a suitably experienced nurse.
6. If you do not know what it is for, leave it turned on; check whether the medical device or piece of equipment is connected to a patient and if that patient appears distressed, report this to a senior nursing colleague straightaway; find out what the medical device is for and any observations you need to make regarding its use.

Activity 10.4: Decision-making (page 175)

You may have included the following points.

1. There were mitigating circumstances (first time doing activity, phone interruption), Tracy's intentions were good, and Robert did not suffer any ill effects; however, not signing a drug chart cannot be justified as it was her duty and not doing so exposed Robert to higher risk.
2. Tracy answered the phone because Robert asked, so she was attentive and accountable to his preferences. However, it was only justifiable if it did not disrupt the intravenous procedure, and we know that it did because she forgot to sign the drug chart.
3. Tracy's possible alternative options: ignore the phone ringing; tell Robert she is sorry but cannot answer it as she needs to finish the procedure (sign chart, dispose of syringe etc.); tell Robert she will answer the phone when she has signed the chart, cleared away and washed hands; if phone is bothering Robert, suggest he tells the caller to ring back later or unplug the phone.
4. Matron was justified because it is better to admit mistakes than cover them up; Robert was entitled to know what happened and to get an apology as stated in *The Code* (*14.2 explain fully and promptly what has happened, including the likely effects, and apologise to the person affected*; NMC, 2015, p12); the medical team also needed to be informed to take any necessary action; it reinforced Tracy's sense of accountability for her actions/omissions; and it facilitated her learning from experience not to repeat the mistake.
5. Three points from NMC (2015, p9) requirements of good record keeping that were not met (any three of the following): *10 Keep clear and accurate records; 10.1 … complete all records at the time; 10.2 identify any risks or problems … so that colleagues who use the records have all the information they need; 10.3 complete all records accurately; 10.4 attribute any entries you make in any paper or electronic records to yourself,*

making sure they are clearly written, dated and timed. If Tracy had signed the drug chart at the time she administered the drug she would not have been distracted from doing so, and her colleagues on the next shift would know the drug had been given and would not have wrongly administered another dose to the patient.

6. It is important that Tracy learns not to make such mistakes because they expose patients to unnecessary risks. She felt it was more by luck than judgement on her part that the outcome was not more serious; other patients might have had a more serious reaction than Robert, and other drugs may be more dangerous if double the prescribed dose is wrongly given.

Further reading

Griffith, R and Tengnah, C (2017) *Law and professional issues in nursing* (4th edn). London: Sage/Learning Matters.

Chapter 3 discusses accountability and professionalism in nursing.

NMC (2015) *Guidance on using social media responsibly.* London: NMC.

Highlights nurses' responsibility not to breach standards set out in *The Code* when using social media.

Peate, I (2016) *The essential guide to becoming a staff nurse.* Chichester: Wiley/Blackwell.

Helpful guide for newly registered nurses and Chapter 4 discusses accountability and delegation.

Useful websites

www.gov.uk/government/publications/the-nhs-constitution-for-england

Department of Health website that shows the latest edition of the NHS Constitution and related documents explaining principles, values and rights/responsibilities of both service users and healthcare workers.

www.nmc-uk.org

NMC website. Click 'About us' then 'Reports and accounts' then 'Fitness to practise annual report' to view reports dating from 2000, or click 'Concerns about nurses and midwives' then 'Attending a hearing' then 'Go to tour' to view an interactive guide to a hearing venue and the roles of those in attendance.

Chapter 11
Confidence in clinical decision-making

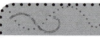

NMC Standards for Pre-registration Nursing Education

This chapter will address the following competencies:

Domain 4: Leadership, management and team working

6. All nurses must work independently as well as in teams. They must be able to take the lead in co-ordinating, delegating and supervising care safely, managing risk and remaining accountable for the care given.

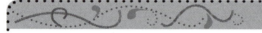

NMC Essential Skills Clusters

This chapter will address the following ESCs:

Cluster: Organisational aspects of care

14. People can trust the newly registered graduate nurse to be an autonomous and confident member of the multidisciplinary or multi-agency team and to inspire confidence in others.

Chapter aims

By the end of this chapter, you should be able to:

*   explain what confidence in decision-making means;
*   relate confidence to your 'three categories of selves';
*   identify what develops or inhibits nurses' confidence;
*   relate confidence to the other perceptions of decision-making;
*   consider how to inspire confidence in patients and healthcare colleagues.

Introduction

In this penultimate chapter of our journey, we conclude the ten perceptions of decision-making by exploring the nature and function of **confidence** when nurses have to make decisions. The NMC emphasises its importance in enabling nurses to be self-directing (autonomous), co-operative and effective healthcare team members. We also need to gain the trust of and inspire confidence in those we care for and work with by being *a model of integrity and leadership* which *should lead to trust and confidence in the profession from patients, people receiving care, other healthcare professionals and the public* (NMC, 2015, p15). If we are not self-directing, we will find it difficult to make our own decisions. If we have problems working as part of a team, we will be less effective in contributing to patients' integrated care pathways. If we cannot get patients to trust us, they will lack confidence in our ability to help them, and feel anxious about their health and wellbeing. Hence, confidence is a vital ingredient nurses need to incorporate in clinical decision-making.

We start by clarifying what confidence in clinical decision-making means. We explore Reinharz's (1997) 'three categories of selves' in relation to our personal and professional (theoretical and practical) self-confidence. We then look at what develops or inhibits confidence in decision-making and explore how confidence is applied within other perceptions of decision-making discussed in this book. Ways of continuing to develop confidence in clinical decision-making after qualifying as a registered nurse are briefly described. The strengths and weaknesses of confidence in decision-making are also outlined. As in previous chapters, case studies and activities are used to engage your interest and assist you in integrating theory and practice.

What is confidence in clinical decision-making?

There are a number of meanings associated with the term 'confidence', as shown below.

1. Trust or belief in a person or thing.
2. Faith in one's own ability; self-assurance.
3. A secret confided to someone.
4. A relationship of mutual trust.
(Chambers, 2016)

All of these meanings are relevant and applied within confidence in clinical decision-making, but they require further clarification. We want patients, clients and other service users to trust us to help them (through safe and effective clinical judgement and decision-making and respecting the confidential nature of their health problems), but in doing so we are morally obliged not to abuse that trust. Confidence tricksters are skilled in soliciting people's trust in order to cheat or harm them in some way, so trusting people and being trusted by others is not necessarily always a good thing. If nurses abuse their privileged position, for example, by stealing from, abusing or sexually assaulting patients, they risk criminal prosecution, being sacked and struck off the NMC register (see Chapter 9). We also have to be aware that some medical conditions, such as toxic confusional states, head injuries, mental disorders and drug dependency can sometimes make it difficult to trust the accuracy of what patients tell us, without carefully checking other sources of evidence.

In other words, developing a trusting relationship is complex – not something we can confirm by ticking a box – and we have to continually work at developing and maintaining trust with patients. As well as trusting others and getting others to trust us, we need to trust in our own abilities. It is necessary to be self-assured in order to have the 'courage of our convictions' and do what we believe to be the right thing. This has been reinforced by the inclusion of 'Courage' in the '6Cs' of compassionate care by nurses and others within the NHS (DH, 2012a). The following case study describes how a new nursing student's lack of self-confidence constrains her ability to make quite basic decisions.

Case study: Ask Mum

Amy, aged 18, had recently commenced a nursing preparation programme. She was asked what she understood by decision-making, and what experience she had of it. Amy did not know how to answer the question, so she was asked how she would go about planning a shopping trip. This is what she replied: 'I talk to my mum about everything. If she agrees with it, I will go and do it; if she doesn't, then I rethink it. She doesn't like certain colours on me so I would have to get something that she liked. In fact, she always comes along to do clothes shopping with me.'

The case study suggests that Amy is compliant and totally dependent on her mother, who makes quite basic decisions on her behalf and overrides any expressed preferences. It highlights how our self-confidence as nurses is helped or hindered by previous life experience (or lack of it). It may seem a little worrying to think that patients are entrusting their health and wellbeing to someone who might say to them, 'Wait a minute; I've got to ask Mum.'

On the other hand, overconfidence is a greater problem as we are more likely to overestimate our abilities, resulting in our clinical judgement, decision-making and related actions being unsafe. It may be easier for someone like Amy to increase their self-confidence (as we shall see later) than it is for an overconfident person to rein it in to a more appropriate level. An overconfident student may be over-compensating for a lack of confidence, and it is difficult for them to acknowledge this. It means that they pose more of a risk to patients (e.g. by undertaking activities they are not competent to perform safely without appropriate supervision) than a student who always seeks guidance. Activity 11.1 asks you to put yourself in the shoes of a nurse who is in charge of a clinical unit where an overconfident nursing student is placed.

Imagine you have completed your nursing programme and are awaiting confirmation of your NMC registration. You are working in a clinical area where you have worked for the last three months, and one of two qualified nurses on your shift has reported sick. When the remaining staff nurse has a break you are left in charge of a group of patients with Nathan, a second-year nursing student, to help you. After answering a phone call at the nurses' station you notice that three patients (suffering from diabetes, epilepsy and dementia) and the nursing student are missing. One of the remaining patients tells you they have just left the unit. You go to the door, see them in the corridor and ask Nathan what he thinks he is doing. He replies, 'Chill out! We're just off to the hospital shop for a bit of "retail therapy" to relieve the boredom, and give these guys a bit of exercise.' What would you do to ensure the safety of all the patients you are responsible for? What would you say to Nathan in order for him to understand the inappropriateness of his actions?

Some possible answers can be found at the end of the chapter.

The case study and Activity 11.1 highlight the need to get the balance right between a timid lack of confidence and overconfident bravado. A self-assured nurse is someone patients can trust to help them rather than expose them to unnecessary, potentially high-risk situations, due to misguided decision-making. Nurses are required to *Act without delay if [they] believe that there is a risk to patient safety* (NMC, 2015, p12). Activity 11.1 also shows how self-assurance is needed to be an assertive advocate on behalf of patients when a colleague or anyone else appears to be jeopardising their health and safety. Understanding that some patients are more vulnerable than others requires knowing them as individuals, their health problems, medical conditions and personal circumstances. It requires confidence in our knowledge of evidence-based practice and its effective application. This is where we have to combine self-assurance and professional assurance to inspire patients to trust our decision-making in delivering safe, high quality nursing care. So, for the purposes of this chapter, confidence in decision-making is understood to mean:

self-assurance from previous personal experience or achievements and professional assurance (respecting confidentiality, applying evidence-based practice) to inspire patients to trust you to help them, and enable you to explain, justify and defend your decisions.

Three categories of selves in personal and professional confidence

When we speak of self-confidence, self-assurance or self-awareness, it suggests we have just one 'self'. Reinharz (1997) argues we have many 'selves' and that understanding the different ways they influence our perceptions, beliefs, attitudes and judgement is important. She is not saying that we all have multiple 'Jekyll and Hyde' personalities. Rather, she is saying we have many contrasting strands of thoughts, feelings and experiences woven together, shaping who we are and what we do. Often we are not aware of them or the different ways that they can influence our judgement. Reinharz was concerned that unless researchers have a better psychological understanding of themselves, personal biases and mistaken beliefs remain unchecked. This can result in them misinterpreting the behaviour they are researching, and inaccurate reporting of evidence.

Like researchers, nurses interact with people to find out information that informs future action, so it is equally important for us to be confident in the accuracy of our observations. Applying reflexivity (Chapter 8) can help us to monitor and control our potential biases, which could otherwise distort our understanding of what we think is true. Reinharz identified three categories of selves that can be used to enhance our critical thinking, reflection and reflexivity in this respect.

- *Brought selves* – past experience shapes our understanding.
- *Research-based selves* – scientific evidence shapes our understanding.
- *Situationally created selves* – interacting with others shapes our understanding.

There are many different strands within each of the three categories, which is why they are referred to as 'selves' rather than 'self'. For example: past experience includes happiness and sadness, successes and failures; there are many different types and ways of obtaining evidence; and we interact with various people and social contexts at different (and unique) moments in time. Table 11.1 cross-references Reinharz's selves to nurses' personal and professional confidence.

Table 11.1 shows how Reinharz's three categories of contrasting 'selves' can be used to map and assess how confident we feel as nurses, personally and professionally, in our decision-making. Cross-referencing our personal assumptions with theoretical evidence or practical experience can also challenge potential biases we may bring with us from the past, as the next case study reveals.

Three categories of selves	Personal confidence	Professional confidence
'Brought selves' (PERSONAL)	Personality, life history influences: how we perceive self and others; how accurate or biased our view of the world is; unresolved emotional 'baggage'; past successes and failures; how self-confident we feel meeting people for the first time or dealing with a new challenge.	

'Research-based selves' (THEORETICAL)		University input influences: accessing relevant information; development of critical thinking to evaluate research evidence; understanding health problems and treatment methods; nurses' role in decision-making; reflection in lifelong learning; confidence to articulate views.
'Situationally created selves' (PRACTICAL)		Work-based learning in clinical practice influences: nurses' identity; engaging with patients, team members; applying theory to practice; developing clinical decision-making skills; respecting patients' confidentiality; developing confidence from sense of achievement helping patients.

Table 11.1: Nurses' personal and professional confidence: three categories of selves

Case study: I imagined doctors would be arrogant

Graham is about to complete his nursing programme, mental health pathway. When asked how he perceives nursing now compared to when he began, he said, 'I imagined before I started the programme that the doctors would be quite arrogant, if you like, and difficult, but I found the opposite actually. I found them to be genuinely quite friendly. They came straightaway if we needed them to review a patient, were always interested in discussing diagnoses, treatments and legal issues with us, and gave me useful information and advice about cognitive therapy for my case study.'

The case study shows that our past experience (brought selves) can give rise to biased opinion and attitudes that might be resistant to change. Fortunately, Graham's prejudice was not so fixed, and when he found it was not supported by his clinical experience ('situationally created selves') and that the opposite seemed to be true (doctors he met were friendly, not arrogant), he revised his judgement accordingly. Applying Reinharz's three categories of selves, therefore, increases our reflexivity by checking out assumptions against alternative types and strength of evidence.

Table 11.1 also reinforces how nursing combines both personal and professional (theoretical and practical) development. The personal dimension may not receive as much attention as the other two either at university or in practice settings, but without it how can we feel confident in our decision-making? Theory, research and practical nursing skills that we learn also add to our repertoire of personal experience (brought selves), which influences how self-confident we feel for our next clinical encounter. Ultimately, clinical decision-making and nursing actions affect the *personal* worlds of our patients, so not losing sight of our own personal needs can remind us to be sensitive and responsive to patients' personal preferences. This can be easily overlooked as we develop our 'research-based selves' amid the complexity and technology of twenty-first-century, evidence-based nursing. However, good communication skills, compassion and caring qualities are what patients value the most about nurses (DH, 2012a), so it is important to integrate and apply personal, theoretical and practical aspects in patient-centred care. Table 11.1 shows this can be facilitated by applying Reinharz's three categories of selves (brought, research-based and situationally created) to develop personal and professional confidence in decision-making. Activity 11.2 asks you to use the three categories of selves to assess your own confidence.

Activity 11.2 — *Reflection*

Look at how Table 11.1 describes the relationships between personal and professional confidence and the three categories of selves, and then answer the following.

1. Look at the description of personal confidence in relation to brought selves and rate your own level of confidence in this respect on a scale of 1–10.
2. Look at professional (theoretical) confidence in relation to research-based selves and rate your own level of confidence in this respect on a scale of 1–10.
3. Look at professional (practical) confidence in relation to situationally created selves and rate your own level of confidence in this respect on a scale of 1–10.
4. Which of the above areas do you feel most confident in?
5. How much variation is there in your confidence scores?
6. Which of the above areas do you feel least confident in?
7. What do you feel would help you to increase your confidence?
8. How are you planning to develop your confidence in this area?

As this is for your own reflection and professional development, there is no outline answer given, but you may find it helpful to discuss a possible action plan with someone that you trust.

Activity 11.2 invited you to explore and assess your own levels of personal, theoretical and practical confidence in clinical judgement and decision-making by applying Reinharz's three categories of selves. By honestly self-assessing areas we lack confidence in, we give ourselves an opportunity to do something about it that can benefit us both personally and professionally. We now turn to look at what inhibits and what develops confidence in clinical decision-making.

What inhibits and what develops confidence in clinical decision-making?

In this section we look at personal, theoretical and practical factors that can enable us to gain or lose confidence in our decision-making ability as nurses. Table 11.2 uses extracts from research into nursing students' clinical decision-making (Standing, 2005, 2007, 2010a) for this purpose.

Factors	Inhibiting confidence	Developing confidence
PERSONAL (brought selves)	• lack of relevant experience, e.g. lady had miscarriage, I didn't know what to say, I just felt inadequate • bullied and victimised in past • bereavement, relationship breakdown and ill health	• relevant past experience • advice and encouragement, e.g. manager felt I was ready for nurse training, I thought yes I'm going for it • stable supportive personal relationships, and 'growing up'
THEORETICAL (research-based selves)	• not enough sessions in skills lab plus relevance of lectures to nursing practice not always clear • theory–practice gap, e.g. theory is patient-centred care – but in practice it is often task-orientated • after qualifying less time to read	• presenting seminar to group, e.g. everyone picks apart what you say, I was nervous but grew very confident • teach other students procedures • keep up to date with journals, e.g. I read journals, surprised how much I knew already, I felt more confident
PRACTICAL (situationally created selves)	• not enough nurses on duty, and shortage of the right equipment • stress of meeting health targets • death of patient you cared for • lack of clinical supervision • making mistakes, e.g. patient did not come to harm but could have; I still get upset about it	• using decision-making skills, e.g. you come out of your shell; by being in a situation you learn to deal with it • mentors instill confidence, e.g. mentor said 'tell me what to do' – scary but it made me think how to plan care • being trusted as a team member • delegated responsibilities, e.g. nominated as case conference speaker

Table 11.2: Factors that inhibit or develop confidence in clinical decision-making

Table 11.2 suggests that confidence in clinical decision-making is a balancing act between inhibiting and developmental factors, including personal, theoretical and practical, or a combination thereof. Nurses are not robots; we are people, too. At any time stressful life events such as the death of a loved one can occur, and when this happens it can shake our confidence not just in our private life but also at work. We all react to stress in different ways, and some of us might find it therapeutic to immerse ourselves in work to avoid having to think about such events. We also experience stress at work if clinical demands exceed the capacity of healthcare providers to deal with it safely and effectively. Perceived stress is exacerbated if we make a mistake or a patient we know dies. At such times *we* may need taking care of a bit more, and mentoring or clinical supervision is useful in this respect, if it is available. As students, stress associated with theoretical factors is usually related to passing written assessments. As far as decision-making is concerned, theoretical factors can help to inform evidence-based decisions and explain them. If relevant theory has 'gone over our head' for one reason or another, we are disadvantaged in this respect. We may also have difficulty managing time in order to keep up to date, especially after we have qualified. If this happens, our evidence-based decision-making is 'past its sell-by date'. Activity 11.3 now asks you to relate Table 11.2 to your experience.

Activity 11.3   *Evidence-based practice and research*

The research findings presented in Table 11.2 are from a longitudinal study conducted between 2000 and 2004. Given the time that has passed since then, this activity asks you to check whether it is relevant and applicable to your current practice.

- Do you think the factors inhibiting confidence are still applicable?
- Do you think the factors developing confidence are still applicable?
- What other factors do you think inhibit confidence in decision-making?
- What other factors do you think develop confidence in decision-making?
- Select two factors inhibiting confidence and identify how to weaken their effect.
- Select two factors developing confidence and identify how to strengthen their effect.

As these are for your own consideration, no outline answers are given. It might be an idea to discuss the activity with peer group, work colleagues, mentor or supervisor to check out their views on it.

We now focus on developing confidence. In Table 11.2 personal, theoretical and practical factors associated with developing confidence in decision-making combined supportive and challenging elements.

- *Personal factors* – supportive relationships versus 'growing up'.
- *Theoretical factors* – peer support versus 'picking apart what you say'.
- *Practical factors* – trusted team member versus 'having to deal with situations'.

It seems that if we just have the supportive input, we will not learn to 'stand on our own two feet' in making decisions, dealing with situations and explaining, justifying and defending actions. On the other hand, if we just have the challenging input, it will be more difficult to develop confidence in the absence of any perceived support. Balancing contrasting and complementary supportive and challenging experiences appears crucial in developing confidence in our decision-making ability. Hence, mentoring and supervision needs to balance being supportive and challenging (Standing, 1999). While we are mainly concerned with developing nurses' confidence in clinical decision-making, it can have 'spin-off' effects in our personal lives, too, as the following case study illustrates.

Case study: Confronting messy housemates

Mark, a third-year nursing student, was asked how he had developed personally since starting the nursing programme and whether this influenced his decision-making ability. He replied, 'In the past, quite often something will happen and go by and I become aware that I did not act in the way I wanted to because I wasn't confident enough that my intuition was right. I have noticed a change in myself recently. I feel more confident now and it affects my personal life too. For example, some of my house-mates are not incredibly diligent with their personal hygiene and I let it go by, but it just got worse. It came to a point where I mentioned it to them. I said they could do what they liked in their rooms but the bathroom and kitchen are for all of us to share so we need to keep them clear of mess for each other's sake. I for one was tired of cleaning up other people's mess before I could get on with what I had to do at the end of a shift. Things did get better afterwards. I don't think I could have done that before I started the programme.'

It takes a certain amount of courage to be self-confident and assertive when we need to be, as others seem to 'step over the line' of acceptable behaviour. Mark's statement is decidedly skewed towards challenging (confronting) as opposed to being supportive, but there is a semblance of support for his housemates' alternative lifestyle in saying 'they can do what they like in their rooms'. (He was also asking them to be supportive of his efforts to keep shared areas clean and tidy.) Theoretical factors such as a better understanding of personal hygiene, infection control and food poisoning, and practical factors regarding lack of access or use of basic facilities, may have also informed Mark's assessment of the situation. In this sense, confidence in personal decision-making can combine personal, theoretical and practical factors. The next case study refers to nurses' confidence in clinical decision-making.

Case study: Finding a voice

Sarah, a third-year nursing student, was asked to reflect on how her understanding of clinical decision-making had developed since commencing the nursing programme. She replied: 'As a first year, you are watching everything in the clinical areas and taking it on-board but you have no voice. In the second year, you get a bit braver and voice opinions about patient care, waiting for support, feedback and confirmation: "Was I right to say that?" Then, as a third year, you are more knowledgeable; you know that what you are proposing is sound because it is research-based, that we should be going that way in our decision-making, and the voice comes out.'

In the case study Sarah associated growth in self-confidence with 'finding her voice' in saying what action needs taking and in justifying her decision-making. Sarah alluded to growth in her understanding of clinical practice ('watching everything' and 'taking it on-board') and knowledge of relevant research and how it applied to patient care. In doing so, Sarah integrated personal (brought selves), theoretical (research-based selves) and practical (situationally created selves) factors that develop our confidence in clinical decision-making. In the final case study we revisit Amy (from page 190) and see how her confidence in clinical decision-making has grown.

Case study: Don't let me die

Amy has now completed the nursing programme and is waiting for her NMC registration to come through. She no longer lives with her mum, as she has got married and has a new home. She has been working on night duty in a medical unit for the last two months. Benjamin, aged 72, is treated for congestive cardiac failure (weakened heart does not pump efficiently, associated with oedema – build-up of fluid in ankles or, more dangerously, in lungs) and chest infection. Benjamin has medication to regulate heart function, remove excess fluid and fight infection. In spite of this, he is usually very perky when he sees Amy. He likes to impart 'pearls of wisdom', repeatedly telling Amy that the most common phrases in the English language are 'I wish' and 'If only'.

One night Benjamin complains he cannot breathe properly. Amy sees he has slipped down the bed and repositions him – with help from an HCA – to elevate and support his back. Amy does this to raise the chest, making breathing easier and reducing the risk of fluid settling in the lungs (pulmonary oedema). Amy checks Benjamin's vital signs and that he has had his medication. Later, he wakes other patients by crying out for help. Amy reports to the clinical manager who instructs her to administer oxygen. Initially it seems to help, but then Benjamin complains again. Amy asks the clinical manager if she should call the doctor. The manager tells her they need a good reason to do so and she should try and calm Benjamin down. However, he gets even more distressed and says, 'Don't let me die, Amy.' Amy is sure something is wrong. She examines Benjamin and sees areas of swelling around his chest and neck that crackle and pop when touched. Benjamin says he feels he is being 'strangled' by his own air. Amy decides she needs to call the duty doctor right away, and then informs the clinical manager. The doctor uses a needle to release air trapped under skin (subcutaneous emphysema) that had leaked out of his lungs, and this relieves the symptoms. The duty manager tells Amy she made the right call.

The case study shows how much Amy has grown in confidence since she started the nursing programme. From someone who was dependent on her mum to make everyday decisions for her, she has become autonomous and confident, assessing risks to Benjamin's health, deciding it required urgent medical intervention and calling the doctor out. In doing so she demonstrated that she has undergone considerable personal and professional development in the space of three years. Her self-confidence has increased through what she called 'growing up'. Professional assurance has increased as Amy has made it her business to keep up to date with nursing research, clinical science and how this can be applied to patients in her care. Amy has combined personal and professional confidence in good interpersonal skills with patients and team members. It was Amy that Benjamin trusted to help him when he was distressed about his breathing problem, and she was instrumental in ensuring the outcome was a positive one. In Table 11.3 Amy's confidence in decision-making is mapped against the conceptions of nursing.

Table 11.3 relates the knowledge, skills and attitudes applied by Amy and the confidence she demonstrated in clinical decision-making to the conceptions of nursing. Activity 11.4 asks you to use the same format to map out your confidence in clinical decision-making.

Conceptions of nursing	Confidence in clinical decision-making
Caring	Supportive in trying to relieve Benjamin's discomfort.
Listening and being there	Responsive to Benjamin's calls for help, and attentive.
Practical procedures	Safely lifts and repositions to improve breathing, gives oxygen, observes vital signs, assesses breathing problem.
Knowledge and understanding	Congestive cardiac failure and chest infection nursing care and medical treatment, clinical science, risk assessment.
Communicating	Establishes good rapport with Benjamin, asking him what was worrying him and advocating medical referral on his behalf.
Patience	Perseveres until solution to problem found, not blaming Benjamin for waking patients; waits before calling for doctor.
Teamwork	Works with HCA to reposition Benjamin, reports change in condition to clinical manager, asks duty doctor to attend.
Paperwork and electronic record	Records vital signs, checks medication chart, records changes in Benjamin's condition and corresponding action.
Empathising and non-judgemental	Senses something was wrong: Benjamin was not his usual perky self, and he was very distressed and frightened.
Professional	Prioritises Benjamin's safety, acts autonomously to call duty doctor urgently and is able to justify decision-making.

Table 11.3: Integrating confidence in clinical decision-making and conceptions of nursing

Activity 11.4   *Decision-making*

Look at how Amy's confidence in clinical decision-making was mapped against the conceptions of nursing in Table 11.3. Identify an incident where you had to find the confidence to deal with a clinical situation. Use the same structure to plot your decision-making and

(Continued)

continued . . .

actions. Notice the number and range of knowledge, skills and attitudes you have identi-fied. Does this help you to articulate and justify what you do in clinical practice? Does it help you identify areas you would like to develop?

As this is for your own development no outline answer is given, but it might be useful to discuss your responses with a mentor or supervisor and possibly agree an action plan.

Confidence in all aspects of clinical decision-making

Like accountability (Chapter 10), confidence alone does not tell us how to make decisions, but it enhances every decision we make as we are more effective and patients feel safer if they sense that we are confident in what we are doing. Table 11.4 applies confidence to the other percep-tions of decision-making in this book.

Table 11.4 represents a quick reference guide that summarises what this book is all about. It identifies a wide range of perceptions of clinical judgement and decision-making, and

Decision-making	Examples of applying confidence
Collaborative	Effective consultation, negotiation and co-operation with patients and team.
Observation	Accurately assessing patients' health using all senses, and report concerns.
Systematic	Methodical application of both critical thinking and problem-solving skills.
Standardised	Thorough implementation of NHS Trust procedures and NICE guidelines.
Prioritising	Vigilant, responsive and effective risk assessment and management skills.
Experience and intuition	Intuitively grasping complex situations and how to react to them quickly.
Reflective	Ability to keep clear head, thinking things through and learning from experience.
Ethical sensitivity	Advocate of patients' rights – informed consent, dignity and confidentiality.
Accountability	Able to explain, justify, defend decision-making with reference to evidence.

Table 11.4: Confidence in relation to perceptions of clinical decision-making

examples of skills used to apply them confidently. This will hopefully help you to be more informed and confident in developing and applying these to patients in your care. In the final chapter we combine and apply all ten perceptions of decision-making described in this book when evaluating nursing decisions. Before that, we take a brief look at how you can continue to develop an appropriate level of confidence in your decision-making after becoming a registered nurse.

How to develop confidence in decision-making as a registered nurse

Throughout your nursing programme you will have had personal tutors and clinical mentors who you can talk to about your personal and professional development. Once you are a registered nurse you have far more responsibilities but fewer opportunities to talk to someone about it. If you do not have any means of ongoing support at work, it can be quite daunting and limits what you learn, as discussing events often helps 'the bell to ring' as you begin to understand more. It is, therefore, highly recommended that you receive clinical supervision that can both support and challenge you to continue to develop your confidence in clinical decision-making and your competence as a nurse. According to Proctor (1986), clinical supervision has three functions, which complement the personal and professional (theoretical and practical) aspects of confidence discussed earlier.

1. *Restorative (supportive)* – coping with stress at work (develop personal confidence).
2. *Formative (educational)* – developing knowledge and skills (develop theoretical confidence).
3. *Normative (managerial)* – monitoring quality of clinical practice (develop practical confidence).

As we have seen in this chapter, all three areas are important in developing confidence in clinical decision-making. Given that nursing practice, healthcare and the nature of health and illness is constantly changing, we need to engage in lifelong learning just to keep up with it. Clinical supervision can make a very useful contribution in this respect, as a way of continuing to develop personal and professional confidence in our nursing competence, judgement and decision-making.

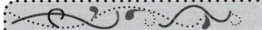

Chapter summary

This chapter explored the concept of confidence and applied it to clinical decision-making in nursing. A distinction was made between self-confidence and inspiring professional confidence in others, such as patients and team members. It was argued that both are needed since clinical decision-making requires self-assurance or assertiveness but also evidence-based knowledge and practical skills to inspire patients to trust us with

(Continued)

continued . . .

their care. Reinharz's three categories of selves (brought, research-based, situationally created) were related to personal, theoretical and practical confidence, and highlighted possible personal biases that need to be challenged. Factors that inhibit or develop confidence in clinical decision-making were identified with reference to research evidence. Case studies were used to demonstrate a progression in students' confidence over a three-year period, and showed how personal, theoretical and practical factors were integrated. Confidence was related to all the other perceptions of decision-making discussed in the book. The strengths of confidence in clinical decision-making include nurses': (i) commitment in making the best evidence-based decisions to enhance patients' health and wellbeing; and (ii) courage to advocate on behalf of our patients. The weaknesses of confidence in clinical decision-making include: (i) lack of confidence where we know the right thing to do but lack the courage to do it; and (ii) over-confidence where we lack insight into the limitations of our competence, resulting in us making errors of judgement and poor decisions that put patients' health and wellbeing at risk. A case was made for the importance of clinical supervision to support, challenge and help us continue our lifelong learning in professional and personal development after qualifying as a nurse.

Activities: brief outline answers

Activity 11.1: Leadership and management (page 191)

You may have included the following points.

Ensuring safety of all patients:

- Instruct Nathan to return to the unit with the three patients immediately.

Talking to Nathan about behaviour:

- He exposed his three patients to unnecessary risks and if anything happened, such as one of them having a fit, or wandering off, he would not be able to cope.
- He exposed the remaining patients in the unit to risk because of the reduced staff numbers.
- He should never take patients out without permission.
- He should always report when he is leaving the unit.

Further reading

Ellis, P and Bach, S (2015) *Leadership, management and team working in nursing* (2nd edn). London: Sage/Learning Matters.

Useful information on clinical supervision, work-based learning environment and leadership role.

Van Ooijen, E (2013) *Clinical supervision made easy: a creative and relational approach for the helping professions* (2nd edn). Monmouth: PCCS Books.

An insightful and practical 3-step guide describing the process and potential benefits of clinical supervision.

Useful website

www.healthwatch.co.uk/rights

Website of the consumer rights watchdog for healthcare listing eight patient rights including *A safe and dignified quality service* and *To be listened to* that nurses and other healthcare workers need to address to inspire confidence in service users.

Chapter 12
Matrix decision-making model and PERSON evaluation tool

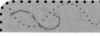

NMC Standards for Pre-registration Nursing Education

This chapter will address the following competencies:

Domain 3: Nursing practice and decision-making
10. All nurses must evaluate their care to improve clinical decision-making, quality and outcomes, using a range of methods, amending the plan of care, where necessary, and communicating changes to others.

Domain 4: Leadership, management and team working
2. All nurses must systematically evaluate care and ensure that they and others use the findings to help improve people's experience and care outcomes and to shape future services.

NMC Essential Skills Clusters

This chapter will address the following ESCs:

Cluster: Care, compassion and communication
5. People can trust the newly registered graduate nurse to engage with them in a warm, sensitive and compassionate way.

Cluster: Organisational aspects of care
10. People can trust the newly registered graduate nurse to deliver nursing interventions and evaluate their effectiveness against the agreed assessment and care plan.

Chapter aims

By the end of this chapter, you should be able to:

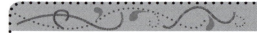

- apply the Matrix model's perceptions of decision-making and conceptions of nursing in reviewing your interventions with patients in clinical practice;
- summarise the main strengths and limitations of the Matrix model of decision-making in nursing;

- understand the importance of evaluating decisions and actions, and being able to demonstrate this;
- describe how a PERSON evaluation tool can be applied to guide and evaluate nursing decisions;
- summarise the main strengths and limitations of PERSON in relation to health policy, *The Code* (NMC, 2015), decision theory and Matrix model of decision-making;
- consider using Matrix model and PERSON to guide, describe and evaluate future decision-making.

Introduction

In this final chapter we draw together all the perceptions of decision-making and conceptions of nursing that have been discussed in the book. We will reflect on ways in which our conceptual understanding of nursing can be applied to practice via the different perceptions of decision-making identified in the **Matrix model**. We will also consider its relevance in light of the continually changing context of healthcare and the challenges this poses. The strengths and weaknesses of the Matrix model of decision-making in nursing are reviewed and a case is made for the development of a complementary, practical guide and evaluation tool.

We then look at the importance of evaluating, learning from and improving our decisions, regardless of which decision theory or perceptions of decision-making we might be applying. A definition of evaluating nursing decisions is presented followed by a **PERSON evaluation tool** which was created by the author to address all the points in the definition. PERSON is described in relation to standards in *The Code* (NMC, 2015) that it incorporates, plus a set of questions testing how person-centred and effective nursing decisions and actions were, and how they can be improved. The strengths and weaknesses of PERSON are identified in relation to: cognitive continuum theory; four decision-making criteria; health policy; *The Code*; and Matrix model of decision-making. Case studies, depicting a patient's observations and experiences of care, are used to show how the Matrix model and PERSON evaluation tool can be applied to practice. Finally, you are invited to consider applying the Matrix model and PERSON in your continuing practice to guide, explain, evaluate and develop your decision-making skills.

Applying the Matrix model of decision-making to everyday nursing practice

The definitions of nursing, clinical judgement and clinical decision-making used in Chapter 1 demonstrated the varied and complex nature of nurses' decisions and related actions or interventions. The Matrix model with its ten perceptions of decision-making and ten conceptions of nursing was proposed as a framework to explore, describe and understand the different processes which underpin our decisions as nurses. Potentially, there are 100 (10 × 10) possible interrelationships between perceptions of decision-making and conceptions of nursing. This illustrates the diverse nature of nursing and the different challenges we face in applying our professional judgement to inform and review what we do as nurses. In order to break this down into manageable chunks, Chapters 2–11 explored each perception of decision-making (and their interrelationships with ten conceptions of nursing) one at a time. In practice, nurses combine all of the perceptions of decision-making and conceptions of nursing every day.

Having examined each perception of decision-making individually, we can now look at how they are applied in various combinations according to patients' needs, clinical context and levels of nursing expertise. The following case study is a patient's observations and reflection on the challenges posed by another patient, and it serves to link different perceptions of decision-making and conceptions of nursing to clinical practice.

> ## Case study: 'I need the ladies!' – Annie's observations of Agnes's care
>
> *I heard a soft but persistent whimpering coming from the bed diagonally opposite to mine. It was evening visiting hour and I could see an elderly man in a chair by the patient's bedside. He was speaking in a soothing voice but one could not miss the slight tone of exasperation in his voice: '… but you have a catheter in, just have a wee.' He was rewarded with a series of pitiful, high-pitched cries and the barely intelligible words, '… but I need the ladies!' The gentleman looked over to me and made an apologetic sign to indicate lack of understanding on the part of the patient who, I assumed, was his wife. The bell rang to mark the end of visiting. The patient in the bed opposite mine explained that the crying was continuous. No one as yet had been able to explain successfully to Agnes, who had just had her right leg amputated above the knee, that she had a catheter fitted or what that meant. Up until the lights were turned off and the ward's inhabitants were settled for the night, the pleading and whimpering continued on and off.*
>
> *The handover took place and the day shift bustled about with routine tasks. The new staff members all had a go at trying to get Agnes to understand her situation but the crying and heart-rending begging went on. Then the miracle happened. The staff nurse who had been administering medications with a cheery smile, speaking to each patient by name, came into the ward along with an HCA and a cardboard bedpan. They drew Agnes's curtains and gave soft-spoken, gentle instructions: 'That's it, Agnes, turn toward me so we can lift your bottom. Good, now turn toward Tina. Yes, good girl, give us a call when you're done.' Blissfully, I listened to minutes of silence until a cheery voice, which I hadn't heard up until now, called out 'Finished!' When the HCA drew back the curtains the staff nurse was just tucking the covers comfortably round Agnes whose eyes were closed now with a peaceful expression on her elderly face. From then on Agnes was brought a bedpan whenever she requested one. I felt her need had at last been successfully met.*

The case study demonstrates that nurses are not alone in making observations and a patient's view of another patient's care reveals how it can affect others in the clinical setting. It also shows how difficult it can be to find the right solution to a problem that was upsetting for Agnes, her husband and the other patients. Activity 12.1 asks you to identify the different perceptions of decision-making alluded to in the case study with reference to any conceptions of nursing that appeared to support the decisions and actions taken.

Activity 12.1 — *Critical thinking and decision-making*

Matrix model template: to identify perceptions of decision-making and conceptions of nursing, showing the interrelationships between them, in relation to an example of clinical decision-making in nursing

Perceptions of decision-making	Conceptions of nursing									
	Caring	Listening and being there	Practical procedures	Knowledge and understanding	Communicating	Patience	Team work	Paperwork and electronic record	Empathising and non-judgemental	Professional
Collaborative										
Observation										
Systematic										
Standardised										
Prioritising										
Experience and intuition										
Reflective										
Ethical sensitivity										
Accountability										
Confidence										

(Continued)

continued . . .

Read through the case study again. Use the Matrix model template on page 207 to map perceptions of decision-making you associate with the nurse's intervention together with the conceptions of nursing that you think were applied. Simply tick the boxes to show interrelationships between 'decision-making' rows and 'nursing' columns and then write brief notes underneath the template explaining the reasons for your selection supported by case study evidence. For example, if we were mapping the other nurses' unsuccessful attempts to communicate with Agnes we could link Observation to: Practical procedures (as it is evident that a urethral catheter is in situ); plus, Knowledge and understanding (urine continually drained from the bladder into a bag via catheter); plus, Communicating (nurses explaining this to Agnes when she kept asking to 'wee' in the toilet); plus, Patience with Agnes (when she fails to understand that she does not need to sit on the toilet to 'wee').

Some possible answers are included at the end of the chapter.

Given the different, contrasting approaches and outcomes described in the case study, your representation of the staff nurse's decision-making and intervention is likely to be different from that of her colleagues. By including all the perceptions of decision-making and conceptions of nursing the Matrix model template can accommodate a wide range of different nursing decisions and actions. Being asked to 'tick boxes' in Activity 12.1 may not seem to be very meaningful. However, it offers a quick way to identify decision-making processes used by nurses and how they incorporate their understanding of nursing in this. It will also provide a pictogram illustrating which perceptions of decision-making were applied more than others. This can be helpful for reflection purposes, for example, were the unused perceptions of decision-making not appropriate, or if they were is there a need for nurses to develop skills in order to apply them? Activity 12.2 invites you to reflect on your clinical practice in this respect.

Activity 12.2   *Reflection, decision-making and critical thinking*

Take time to reflect upon any recent clinical experience, trying to identify examples of the perceptions of decision-making and conceptions of nursing that were applied. Use the above Matrix model template to map interrelationships between perceptions of decision-making and conceptions of nursing. Write a brief description explaining how the perceptions of decision-making and corresponding conceptions were applied in the clinical experience. Why did you choose this example of clinical experience? Is it an example of effective decision-making with a successful outcome, or less effective decision-making with an unsuccessful outcome? Looking back, does the pattern of decision-making perceptions and nursing conceptions you identified help to explain what occurred? Are there any other perceptions of decision-making and conceptions

continued . . .

of nursing, not applied at the time, which may have resulted in a better outcome? Having worked through this learning activity, are there any perceptions of decision-making you want to develop your skills in? How will you go about doing so?

As this activity is for your own reflective learning and development, there is no outline answer provided.

Strengths and weaknesses of the Matrix model of decision-making

The Matrix model offers a comprehensive overview of the knowledge, skills, attitudes and values associated with nurses in addressing patients', clients' and service users' healthcare needs and preferences. As such, it conveys nurses' unique professional identity by showing how we integrate personal (embodied), practical (embedded) tacit knowledge with theoretical, research-based explicit knowledge and ethical values. All of this informs our clinical judgement, decision-making and nursing interventions. The Matrix model reflects and assists in promoting the '6Cs': care, compassion, competence, communicating, courage and commitment, and their application within collaborative, patient-centred, evidence-based care (DH, 2012a). As demonstrated throughout this book, the Matrix model also complements the NMC *Standards for pre-registration nursing education* and the standards of practice and behaviour set out in *The Code* (NMC, 2010, 2015).

Complementary and contrasting decision-making processes are incorporated within the Matrix model (e.g. experiential and intuitive, collaborative and reflective practice, prioritising and risk management, systematic and standardised evidence-based practice, and ethical sensitivity and accountability). This offers nurses a wide-ranging 'toolkit' to tackle patients' diverse physical and psychological health issues. For example, in the case study the scientifically informed systematic and standardised approach, so necessary in surgical procedures and post-operative wound care, was ineffective in resolving Agnes's psychological needs. It is therefore advisable not to get stuck in one particular mode of decision-making because different patients with different problems will require adjustments in the approach taken. This is consistent with cognitive continuum theory (Chapter 1) which recommends flexibility in how intuitive or analytical our decisions need to be, in order to match them to the particular demands and context of situations we have to deal with.

The weaknesses of the Matrix model are in a way the 'flip side' of its strengths. Its comprehensive overview of decision-making in nursing means that each approach referred to could be explored in greater depth (as indeed they are elsewhere; Standing, 2010a, 2010b). Similarly, its broad focus in appealing to the four nursing pathways (adult, child, mental health and learning disability) in pre-registration education may require supplementing with additional pathway-specific examples of decision-making. The four-year longitudinal hermeneutic phenomenological research study of nursing students' developmental journey in acquiring decision-making skills, culminating in the creation of the Matrix model, was completed in 2005. The continuing relevance of the Matrix model cannot, therefore, be taken for granted. Case studies from the original research have been supplemented with more recent examples that serve to demonstrate its continuing relevance in explaining clinical judgement and decision-making in nursing. This is helped by a caring and collaborative characterisation of nursing that is endorsed by *The Code* and current health policy.

While the Matrix model provides a comprehensive framework to describe nurses' decisions, it can be time consuming to go through all of the different permutations when caring for a patient in a busy clinical area. With this in mind a complementary PERSON evaluation tool, derived from the Matrix model, was created. It presents an accessible framework to both guide and evaluate decision-making. We will explore this in more detail after clarifying what we mean by evaluating nursing decisions.

What does 'evaluating nursing decisions' mean?

To evaluate means *to form an idea or judgement about the worth of something* or *to calculate the value of something* (Chambers, 2016). The 'something' we are concerned with is nurses' clinical decision-making, as defined in Chapter 1. Evaluating nursing decisions is vital because we need to know whether our actions have been effective in promoting patients' health, recovery from illness or relief of suffering. If there is no improvement, we need to review whether we have carried out procedures properly or reconsider the plan of care. Continually evaluating decisions is essential in order to ensure that nursing interventions address patients' individual and changing needs. Evaluation is a key part of the nursing process. This chapter argues that all nursing decisions need to be evaluated, in addition to those where the nursing process has been applied.

Evaluating nursing decisions can be complex and challenging because it requires us to be quite detached in making an objective judgement about the quality of our own clinical judgement/decision-making in caring for patients. In Chapter 4 we noted that evaluation (critiquing things) is the highest of six levels of critical thinking used to review nursing interventions and revise plans as needed. In Chapter 8, we noted that reflexivity, the critical self-examination of ideas, assumptions and biases, is a more inward-looking form of evaluation to improve the accuracy and effectiveness of nurses' perceptions, judgement and decision-making. Evaluating nursing decisions, therefore, requires inward and outward application of critical thinking skills to examine ourselves as well as our patients' response to healthcare interventions.

As a nurse, it can be difficult to face or accept criticism if you feel you have done the best you can to help a patient in challenging circumstances. This is a natural reaction, but as accountable professionals we have to 'swallow our pride', learn from mistakes and improve our knowledge and skills so we can be better nurses. We also need to 'celebrate our success' where we made the right decision and carried out care skilfully, which patients benefited from and were satisfied with. In this way, evaluating nursing decisions contributes to the development of good practice and the particular knowledge, skills and attitudes associated with it.

For the purposes of this book evaluating nursing decisions is defined as follows:

a critical review of nursing decisions and associated care in: (i) addressing patients' rights, needs, problems and preferences; (ii) avoiding causing harm to patients; (iii) carrying out interventions that have beneficial outcomes for patients; (iv) applying relevant evidence, research and clinical guidelines to patient care; (v) identifying strengths and weaknesses of care provided; and (vi) considering the implications of the findings for continuing patient care and our own professional development and education needs as nurses.

Developing a PERSON evaluation tool

The above definition is quite long because nursing is a complex process, and it follows that nurses' decision-making and related actions are multifaceted. Given the enormous range of nursing decisions, how can we come up with a method of evaluation that is universally applicable?

We can begin to develop a guide to evaluate nursing decisions by picking out points from the definition, and asking questions to test them. For example, the definition refers to *patients' rights, avoiding causing harm, beneficial outcomes* and *applying relevant evidence*. These are important points to consider in developing a guide to evaluate nursing decisions. The first three were explored in Chapter 9, and the remaining chapters have explored different kinds of evidence and ways of applying it within the other nine perceptions of decision-making. The central focus of respecting patients' human rights and treating them as equal partners in decisions about their care provides the inspiration for calling the evaluation tool PERSON. This echoes healthcare policy priorities in: fostering a patient-centred culture of compassionate care; improving the safety, effectiveness and quality of healthcare; maximising potential beneficial outcomes, and patients' experience of care (DH, 2012a, 2012b, 2013a, 2016b). The next case study offers an insight into a patient's experience where compassionate care was sometimes secondary to completing certain tasks.

Case study: I wanted to shout, 'I'm here! It's me – Annie!'

The first person one communicates with through a verbal exchange, or just a meeting of the eyes, entirely colours the moment. So, if that person is a doctor on rounds, or a nurse with medication, or an HCA with blood pressure machine in hand, the vital aspect of this first encounter upon awakening is whether it conveys warmth, kindness – a shared humanity. However, if the staff member is focused on accomplishing a set of tasks and recording the results, the risk is that a gulf, empty of empathy, looms wide between them. And yet, that risk can be so easily mitigated or even eliminated by the staff member addressing you by your first name: Annie, how are you feeling today? Or: Annie, I have your medication here. Or: Annie, can I just take your blood pressure? Failing that, meeting a staff member's eyes and seeing friendliness there or catching a gentle smile can in an instant turn a fearful, confusing moment into a calming, reassuring one.

(Continued)

continued . . .

Can it really make so much difference to the patient experience? The answer is a simple 'Yes!' – all the difference. After two major operations and nearly 4 weeks on the 'step down' ward from intensive care, where I had two separate stays of 3 days each, it would be churlish of me to fault the care I received from so many competent professionals in the health service. What is starkly vivid in my mind, however, are those instances when, upon awakening, the person tending to me was, for example, either concentrating fixedly on what they were doing or, perhaps, calling out to someone else on the ward, but certainly not interacting in any way, shape or form with me. On those few occasions I felt demeaned instantly by those members of staff. I became a non-person, a slab of humanity on a mattress. I registered not just their indifference to my vulnerability but a total blindness to my identity. I wanted to shout, 'I'm here! It's me – Annie!'

The case study suggests that while Annie's physical needs appeared to be addressed satisfactorily through the systematic delivery of standardised procedures and observations, her psychological wellbeing was sometimes overlooked when those attending to various tasks did not engage with her. This echoes some students' criticisms in linking standardised care plans to task orientated care (Chapter 5). It suggests that healthcare staff were not adequately addressing Annie's right of self-determination (Chapter 9) or her need to communicate and 'connect' to enhance her sense of wellbeing (Roper et al., 2000; Aked et al., 2008). Integrating ethical sensitivity, collaborative and reflective decision-making with standardised procedures would help ensure nurses and other healthcare workers offer more person-centred, holistic and humane care.

Annie is an observant, thoughtful, sensitive and articulate person and yet she was made to feel at times that she was *a non-person, a slab of humanity on a mattress.* This is very similar to the way many people with learning disabilities feel in not being accepted as human beings in their own right. When Annie wanted to shout, 'I'm here! It's me – Annie!' she expressed the same sentiment as Mencap (voluntary body committed to securing equal opportunities and social inclusion for people with learning disabilities) in their 'Here I am: Understand me' campaign, that promotes understanding and acceptance of people with learning disabilities. Clearly it is not right for anyone to be made to feel that they are a non-person, especially when they are in a healthcare setting that is supposed to promote, restore and enhance their health and sense of wellbeing.

In revising *The Code*, the NMC presents standards of practice and behaviour under four headings: *prioritise people, practise effectively, preserve safety* and *promote professionalism and trust*. It reflects concerns that these qualities have been lacking, and recommendations that they must be prioritised. Healthcare professionals must be open and honest in acknowledging and learning from mistakes, and take action to improve their practice (Francis Report, 2013; Keogh Report, 2013). It also reinforces our duty to respect people's human rights by working in partnership with them to address their healthcare needs, as opposed to doing things to them. In total there are 25 standards and 109 related competencies in *The Code* under the four headings (NMC, 2015). Ultimately, every nursing decision and intervention we make must comply with the NMC *Code*. This was underlined in Chapter 10 where we noted that some nurses had been struck off the NMC register for seriously breaching *The Code*. It is important that all nurses and midwives are familiar with *The Code* and comply with its standards. In practical terms it is not possible to run through such an extensive checklist when evaluating decisions. We therefore need to create a more concise form of words that focuses on essential points in evaluating nursing decisions whilst echoing key requirements of *The Code*. With this in mind, the PERSON evaluation tool combines aspects of the Matrix model with selected professional standards (NMC, 2015).

PERSON acronym	Relevant extracts from *The Code* (NMC, 2015)
P PERSON-centred *[prioritise people]*	• *Listen to people and respond to their preferences and concerns* (p4) • *Make sure that people's physical, social and psychological needs are assessed and responded to* (p5) • *Make sure that you get properly informed consent and document it before carrying out any action* (p6) • *Respect people's right to privacy and confidentiality*
E EVIDENCE-based *[practise effectively]*	• *Always practise in line with the best available evidence* (p7) • *Make sure that any information or advice given is evidence-based, including information relating to using any healthcare products or services* • *Maintain the knowledge and skills you need for safe and effective practice* • *Take account of current evidence, knowledge and developments in reducing mistakes and the effect of them* (p14)
R RISKS assessed and managed	• *Work with colleagues to preserve the safety of those receiving care* (p8) • *Identify any risks or problems that have arisen and the steps taken to deal with them, so that colleagues who use the records have all the information they need* (p9) • *Act without delay if you believe that there is a risk to patient safety or public protection* (p12) • *Take all reasonable personal precautions necessary to avoid any potential health risks to colleagues, people receiving care and the public* (p14)
S SAFE and effective delivery of care *[preserve safety]*	• *Recognise and work within the limits of your competence* (p11) • *Make a timely and appropriate referral to another practitioner when it is in the best interests of the individual needing any action, care or treatment* • *Ask for help from a suitably qualified and experienced healthcare professional to carry out any action or procedure that is beyond the limits of your competence* • *Stay objective and have clear professional boundaries at all times with people in your care (including those who have been in your care in the past), their families and carers* (p15)

(Continued)

Table 12.1: (Continued)

PERSON acronym	Relevant extracts from *The Code* (NMC, 2015)
O OUTCOMES of care benefit patient	• *Recognise when people are anxious or in distress and respond compassionately and politely* (p5) • *Act in partnership with those receiving care, helping them to access relevant health and social care, information and support when they need it* • *Keep clear and accurate records relevant to your practice* (p9) • *Confirm that the outcome of any task you have delegated to someone else meets the required standard* (p10)
N NURSING and midwifery strengths and weaknesses identified and acted upon to improve practice *[promote professionalism and trust]*	• *Work with colleagues to evaluate the quality of your work and that of the team* (p8) • *Gather and reflect on feedback from a variety of sources, using it to improve your practice and performance* • *Be open and candid with all service users about all aspects of care and treatment, including when any mistakes or harm have taken place* (p11) • *Use all complaints as a form of feedback and an opportunity for reflection and learning to improve practice* (p18)

Table 12.1: PERSON: Clinical decision-making evaluation tool – Part A

The PERSON acronym in Table 12.1 reinforces the importance of respecting patients' and service users' rights as unique individuals with specific needs and preferences, and treating them with dignity in dealing with their problems. Each letter of PERSON focuses upon an area to evaluate, and collectively they cover all the points referred to in the definition of evaluating nursing decisions. These six areas are also representative of key sections within *The Code* (NMC, 2015) and relevant extracts are included to highlight this. Table 12.1 (Part A) offers a general template in evaluating nursing decisions with reference to *The Code*. Table 12.2 (Part B) replaces extracts from the NMC *Code* with probing questions to test the extent to which PERSON evaluation criteria have been addressed.

Together, Parts A and B of PERSON offer a concise overview of key considerations in the provision and evaluation of high quality, patient-centred, evidence-based decision-making and nursing care. This is a universal tool that can be applied to adult, mental health, learning disability and child nursing pathways, and to midwifery (nurses and midwives are professional 'siblings' governed by the same *Code)*. Knowing that your decisions and interventions need to be evaluated means it is important to incorporate PERSON criteria when planning and implementing care. Different pathways deal with different sorts of problems, applying different sorts of knowledge and skills. So it may need supplementing with pathway-specific decision tools reflecting the different evidence base and risk assessment tools applied.

The last section of PERSON, Nursing and midwifery strengths and weaknesses, facilitates being honest with ourselves to address our professional development needs, and to enhance the quality

PERSON acronym	Answer questions to evaluate decisions
P PERSON-centred *[prioritise people]*	Were different care options explained to the patient? Did the patient give consent before the intervention? How did the patient's opinion contribute to care plans? If for any reason the patient was unable to contribute to decisions, how were his or her rights safeguarded?
E EVIDENCE-based *[practise effectively]*	What patient observations indicated a need for action? What corroborating evidence supports your assessment? What was the rationale for the selected intervention? What research evidence underpins the intervention?
R RISKS assessed and managed	What threats to patient's health/wellbeing were there? What was done to ensure a safe healthcare environment? What procedure did you follow to control known risks? How did you escalate concerns if problems worsened?
S SAFE and effective delivery of care *[preserve safety]*	What knowledge/skills/attitudes were applied to care? What prior experience did you have of this intervention? How was your competence to give care quality assured? How did you share information on the care you gave?
O OUTCOMES of care benefit patient	What was the patient's/relatives' feedback about care? To what extent were desired outcomes of care achieved? How do you think the patient benefited from this care? How will you address any negative outcomes of care?
N NURSING and midwifery strengths and weaknesses identified and acted upon to enhance practice *[promote professionalism and trust]*	What did you learn from this episode of patient care? How did you justify public trust in your ability to care? On reflection, what could you have done differently? What are you doing to improve decision-making skills?

Table 12.2: PERSON: Clinical decision-making evaluation tool – Part B

of care we give. The importance of honesty, openness, candour and integrity was emphasised in the Francis Report and is reflected in *The Code*. If we remain unaware of things we need to improve or choose not to do anything about them, it will stunt our professional growth and limit our effectiveness as nurses. If we were to go one step further down this 'slippery slope' and make false claims in order to cover up errors or omissions in care, it amounts to dishonesty. This would be a serious breach of *The Code* (NMC, 2015), which could put our jobs and our registration as nurses in jeopardy. It is therefore better for our patients and ourselves if we are open and honest in reflecting upon and evaluating our practice. Applying the PERSON evaluation tool helps us do this and provides evidence that we are committed to lifelong learning to review and improve our nursing skills. It is therefore recommended that you use Parts A and B of PERSON as a checklist to guide and evaluate your clinical decisions and actions.

Applying the PERSON evaluation tool to review nursing decisions and actions

In order to show how PERSON can be applied to enhance decision-making in nursing, a case study is presented to identify strengths and weaknesses of nurses' decision-making and care. It is the third and final instalment of Annie's observation and reflection upon her recent stay in an acute hospital setting. As such it offers a certain authenticity in representing patients' experiences which healthcare professionals are obliged to be attentive and responsive to. Again it is focused upon adult pathway care, but it is hoped that the issues raised have parallels with other pathways and that it is possible to transfer learning to nursing in alternative clinical settings.

> ## Case study: How to (or not to) prioritise people and practise effectively
>
> *The sister came into the ward around 11.00 am and went straight to Rosemary who was sitting reading in a chair next to her bed: 'We're going to give you the enema this afternoon just after lunch and then you'll be taken down to X-ray.' 'Oh dear, please, no,' replied a clearly distressed Rosemary. 'Yes, Rosemary, you were told yesterday by the consultant that you would have to have the enema before the radiologist takes some pictures; otherwise we can't find out what's wrong with you. Don't you want to get rid of the pain and get better?' 'Yes, of course I do, but I don't want to have an enema, I really don't.' 'Now, let's not be difficult, Rosemary, there's nothing to it. Patients have them every day. You had it all explained to you yesterday,' responded the sister, with poorly hidden irritation in her voice. She then walked out of the ward.*
>
> *The staff nurse, who was dispensing medications from the trolley in the next bay, glanced over towards Rosemary, who was shaking slightly now and one or two tears slipped down her pale cheeks. She reached for a white lace hanky from the drawer and quietly wiped away the tears. The staff nurse finished making a note of the medication she had just dispensed, locked up the drugs trolley and went over to Rosemary, who was clutching the hanky tightly in her lap. The staff nurse dropped down to a crouch, took Rosemary's hands in both of hers, and just held them without saying a word. After a few moments Rosemary murmured, 'I'm just so frightened.' The nurse nodded gently and said softly, 'I know.' 'What if I have an accident? What if I can't hold it in,' she pleaded quietly, gazing down into the nurse's eyes? 'It sometimes happens. It doesn't matter. We'll give you a little rest and just try it again.' The two figures stayed still in the same positions. After a moment or two, Rosemary made a final wipe of her cheeks with the hanky and gave the nurse a weak smile. The staff nurse gave Rosemary's hands a last quick squeeze, stood up and pushed the drugs trolley out of the ward.*

The case study reveals two different approaches in dealing with Rosemary's resistance and fear of being given an enema in preparation for radiological investigation of her gastrointestinal problem. It helps to highlight the challenges of being patient-centred (prioritise people) and efficient in carrying out procedures to enable healthcare colleagues to accurately diagnose and treat medical problems (practise effectively).

The sister's approach was not person-centred or collaborative. She simply told Rosemary what was going to happen and why it was necessary, dismissed her anxiety and concerns about this and accused her of being 'difficult' when Rosemary said, 'I don't want to have an enema'. The outcome of the sister's intervention was that Rosemary was upset, tearful and fearful of the impending procedure.

The staff nurse's approach was person-centred and collaborative. She intuitively used the evidence of her senses to observe Rosemary was upset, and used 'listening and being there' skills to enable her to express fears about the enema. She was patient, compassionate and caring and communicated this to Rosemary verbally and non-verbally, and demonstrated ethical sensitivity, empathy and a non-judgemental attitude in doing so. She prioritised Rosemary's care to minimise risks to her psychological wellbeing, and applied her knowledge and skills very competently in providing high quality, safe and effective care. The outcome of the staff nurse's intervention was that Rosemary stopped crying, felt comforted, was able to voice her concerns about the procedure, was reassured that she would be taken care of and no longer said she did not want an enema. It is an excellent example of how to justify public trust in nurses' professionalism.

Activity 12.3   *Critical thinking and decision-making*

This activity focuses upon identifying weaknesses and improving them. Read through the above case study again. Go back to Table 12.1: 'PERSON: Clinical decision-making evaluation tool – Part A', look at each section, and

- identify any extracts of the NMC *Code* which, based on the case study evidence presented, did not appear to be complied with;
- identify any mitigating factors that may have contributed to this non-compliance;
- suggest ways in which the person concerned could be helped to comply with these standards in future;
- explain what might be the consequences of either not being aware of one's non-compliance or having been made aware of it, not changing one's practice and behaviour accordingly.

Some possible answers can be found at the end of the chapter.

Matrix model of decision-making and PERSON evaluation tool

Table 12.3 shows how different combinations of the perceptions of decision-making and conceptions of nursing within the Matrix model relate to the six different elements of PERSON. For example, the previous case study showed how 'collaborative' clinical decision-making involves 'listening and being there' and 'empathising and non-judgemental' conceptions of nursing in giving person/patient-centred care. Hence, the PERSON evaluation tool offers a framework in which the Matrix model can be applied in guiding, understanding, explaining and evaluating

PERSON acronym	Perceptions of decision-making	Conceptions of nursing
P PERSON-centred *[prioritise people]*	• Collaborative • Ethical sensitivity • Observation • Accountability	• Listening and being there • Empathising and non-judgemental
E EVIDENCE-based *[practise effectively]*	• Observation • Reflective • Systematic • Standardised	• Knowledge and understanding
R RISKS assessed and managed	• Prioritising • Observation • Systematic • Standardised	• Practical procedures
S SAFE and effective delivery of care *[preserve safety]*	• Experience and intuition • Collaborative • Systematic • Confidence	• Caring • Patience • Teamwork
O OUTCOMES of care benefit patient	• Observation • Reflective • Collaborative • Ethical sensitivity	• Communicating • Paperwork and electronic record
N NURSING and midwifery strengths and weaknesses identified and acted upon to enhance practice *[promote professionalism and trust]*	• Accountability • Ethical sensitivity • Reflective	• Professional

Table 12.3: PERSON evaluation tool and Matrix model of decision-making

nursing decisions. Used together they enable us to *prioritise people, practise effectively, preserve safety* and *promote professionalism and trust* (NMC, 2015), by identifying the knowledge, skills and attitudes needed for effective clinical judgement and decision-making in nursing.

Cognitive continuum decision theory and PERSON evaluation tool

It has been proposed that PERSON is a credible evaluation tool for nursing decisions because: (i) it addresses this book's definition of evaluation; (ii) it addresses key standards of practice and behaviour in *The Code* (NMC, 2015); and (iii) it is derived from research into nurses' perceptions of decision-making (Standing, 2005, 2007, 2010a). We will now see how it 'shapes up' in relation to decision theory. We will do this by mapping the perceptions of decision-making against a cognitive continuum of clinical judgement. We will then apply the criteria of practicality, logic, relevance and rigour (derived from cognitive continuum decision theory) to critique PERSON. As mentioned in Chapter 1, cognitive continuum theory integrates widely contrasting methods of decision-making, ranging from intuitive hunches to the analysis and application of research (Hammond, 1996; Standing, 2010b). It provides a comprehensive overview of different kinds of human judgement and different kinds of research, and how they inform different kinds of decisions. In Figure 12.1, the ten perceptions of decision-making are matched to five modes of clinical judgement within a cognitive continuum.

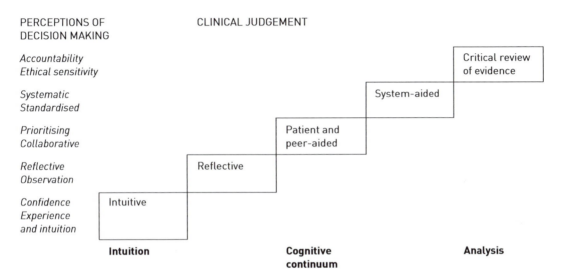

Figure 12.1: A cognitive continuum of five modes of clinical judgement and ten perceptions of decision-making in nursing

Figure 12.1 shows how the ten perceptions of decision-making associated with PERSON (Table 12.3) also correspond to five modes of clinical judgement along a cognitive continuum ranging from intuition to analysis. It indicates that PERSON is a flexible system to review a wide range of decisions and is supported by cognitive continuum theory. As noted in Chapter 1, intuition helps us to quickly sense what we need to do in response to a change in a patient. For example, in the last case study the staff nurse intuitively reacted to Rosemary's state of distress. However, human perception is prone to error and bias, so we might 'misread' a situation. Analysis helps us to be detached and objective and apply research-based evidence to care, and minimise individual errors of judgement. However, research takes time and may not yet have all the answers for understanding or addressing an individual patient's problems. There are more analytical modes than shown in Figure 12.1, but they refer to actually carrying out research studies to inform decisions (Hammond, 1996; Standing, 2010b), which is not a practical option for most nursing decisions. Our evidence-based decision-making mainly draws on and applies research that has

Cognitive continuum criteria	Examples from PERSON evaluation tool – Part B
Practicality – is it achievable?	To what extent were desired outcomes of care achieved?
Logic – is it explainable?	What was the rationale for the selected intervention?
Relevance – is it justifiable?	How did you justify public trust in your ability to care?
Rigour – is it defensible?	What research evidence underpins the intervention?

Table 12.4: Practicality/logic/relevance/rigour and PERSON evaluation tool

already been done, for example, applying NICE clinical practice guidelines (system-aided judgement) within standardised clinical decision-making.

Cognitive continuum theory also identified contrasting criteria with which to assess the quality of any decision: correspondence competence, coherence competence, ecological validity and scientific validity (Hammond, 1996). These have been reworded as: practicality, logic, relevance and rigour (Standing and Standing, 2010). We can assess whether decisions satisfy these criteria by asking specific questions associated with them (as we did in Chapter 1). If applying the PERSON evaluation tool is an effective way to review nursing decisions and interventions, we would expect it to test whether these criteria have been met. We will see whether it does by looking at Table 12.4.

Table 12.4 shows that the PERSON evaluation tool (Part B) includes questions that probe how well nursing decisions satisfy criteria derived from cognitive continuum theory. This reinforces its credibility and usefulness as a tool to evaluate nursing decisions. We now need to check whether it can contribute to a culture of compassionate care.

The PERSON evaluation tool and compassionate care

Health policy requires the '6Cs' of compassionate care (care, compassion, competence, communication, courage, commitment) to be applied *in our everyday care of patients*. It also says we need to *Embed the 6Cs in all nursing and midwifery university education and training* (DH, 2012a). The PERSON evaluation tool relates well to the '6Cs' of compassionate care: 'P' stands for 'person-centred' care that respects individuals' needs and preferences (*compassion*); 'E' stands for 'evidence-based' care, where nurses apply approved interventions (*competence*); 'R' stands for 'risks assessed and managed' that prevents avoidable harm to patients (*care*); 'S' stands for 'safe and effective delivery of care' achieved through a well co-ordinated team effort (*communication*); 'O' stands for 'outcomes of care benefit patient' where we need to be vigilant in monitoring progress (*commitment*); 'N' stands for 'nursing and midwifery strengths and weaknesses identified and acted upon to enhance practice' involving being honest about how we can improve the quality of care that we give to patients (*courage*). In addition:

1. PERSON incorporates key criteria from *The Code* (NMC, 2015), which sets our professional standards in providing high quality, compassionate nursing care.
2. PERSON incorporates conceptions of nursing that closely relate to the '6Cs': *caring, listening and being there, knowledge and understanding, communicating, empathising and non-judgemental* and *professional*.
3. PERSON incorporates perceptions of decision-making that apply compassion to nursing decisions including: *ethical sensitivity, experience and intuition, reflective, collaborative, prioritising* and *accountability*.

The '6Cs' of compassionate care are therefore firmly embedded within the PERSON evaluation tool. As such, PERSON serves as both an educational resource and a practical guide that complements the application of the '6Cs' to patient care. In doing so, it enables nurses to address health policy priorities (DH, 2012a), and incorporate these values within their professional identity. It is recommended that you use this evaluation tool within your Professional Development Portfolio to guide and evaluate your clinical judgement and decision-making and help to address lifelong learning needs, such as NMC revalidation to maintain registered nurse status.

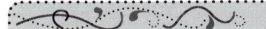

Chapter summary

This chapter revisited the perceptions of decision-making and conceptions of nursing within the Matrix model, and explored how to evaluate nursing decisions and interventions. We began by recognising that nurses use different combinations of the perceptions of decision-making and conceptions of nursing, according to the situations they are faced with and their level of expertise. A main strength of this model was identified as integrating essential nursing knowledge, skills and attitudes in providing a comprehensive understanding of the wide-ranging processes that nurses apply in their decision-making in diverse and challenging clinical settings. Weaknesses were related to its strengths, for example, there are 100 possible interrelationships between decision-making and nursing themes which can limit its practicality in clinical settings. A case was made for incorporating the Matrix model in a more concise form to guide and evaluate decision-making.

We then defined the process of evaluating decisions in nursing contexts. In order to address all the points in the definition a PERSON evaluation tool was presented with six key elements (e.g. P = *Person-centred*, E = *Evidence-based*) to guide and evaluate nursing decisions. We found a close correspondence with, and incorporated key standards from, *The Code* (NMC, 2015) to show how they relate to each element of PERSON. A checklist of questions was developed to test how well nursing decisions and interventions address each aspect of PERSON. We matched the Matrix model's ten perceptions of decision-making

(Continued)

continued . . .

(e.g. *Collaborative*) and ten conceptions of nursing (e.g. *Caring*) to different elements of PERSON. The criteria of practicality, logic, relevance and rigour, derived from cognitive continuum theory to assess the quality of decisions, were shown to be adequately tested by the evaluation tool. Case studies of a patient's recent hospital experiences showed how the Matrix model and PERSON evaluation tool can be used to enhance compassionate care, by nurses matching their decisions and actions to patients' individual needs and preferences.

The main strengths of the PERSON evaluation tool are as follows:

(i) Concise, accessible, coherent, universal framework to systematically guide and evaluate nursing decisions, reflect on results and make improvements as needed;

(ii) Derived from research into nurses' perceptions of decision-making and enables application of the findings, the Matrix model, to practice;

(iii) Applies NMC Standards from *The Code* (*prioritise people, practise effectively, preserve safety, promote professionalism and trust*) in each element of PERSON;

(iv) Enhances nurses' professional identity by integrating a unique mixture of knowledge, skills and values, applied in compassionate, patient-centred, evidence-based care.

A possible weakness of PERSON is that it may need supplementing with pathway-specific decision tools, for example, risk assessment criteria differ from one clinical setting to another. Nevertheless, it is recommended that you consider applying PERSON to guide and evaluate your clinical decisions; in writing your Professional Development Portfolio; and in submitting evidence for NMC revalidation, as necessary.

Activities: brief outline answers

Activity 12.1: Critical thinking and decision-making (pages 207–8)

Mapping perceptions of decision-making and conceptions of nursing the staff nurse applied with Agnes:

It appears that all of the perceptions of decision-making and conceptions of nursing were applied in caring for Agnes. 'Collaborative' was the only perception of decision-making that is interrelated with all the conceptions of nursing and 'Caring' was the only conception of nursing that interrelated with all the perceptions of decision-making. The predominant pattern of the staff nurse's decision-making is therefore collaborative and caring. Although there was no medical reason for Agnes to need a bedpan in order to urinate (due to catheter in situ) the staff nurse provided one because Agnes felt she needed the toilet and was distressed by being told she did not. It is possible that the catheter caused Agnes irritation which she associated with needing to 'wee' on the toilet, as she seemed unaware that she had a catheter fitted. The staff nurse combined patience, caring, listening, communicating and empathising qualities with practical skills and teamwork by enlisting the help of the HCA with the bedpan. While there is no reference to record keeping, we are told that after this incident Agnes was given a bedpan whenever she requested it which suggests the intervention was recorded and incorporated into her plan of care.

Matrix model template: to identify perceptions of decision-making and conceptions of nursing, showing the interrelationships between them, in relation to an example of clinical decision-making in nursing

Conceptions of nursing

Perceptions of decision-making	Caring	Listening and being there	Practical procedures	Knowledge and understanding	Communicating	Patience	Team work	Paperwork and electronic record	Empathising and non-judgemental	Professional
Collaborative	✓	✓	✓	✓	✓	✓	✓	✓	✓	✓
Observation	✓	✓	✓	✓					✓	
Systematic	✓		✓	✓			✓	✓		✓
Standardised	✓		✓							
Prioritising	✓	✓	✓				✓			
Experience and intuition	✓	✓	✓	✓	✓	✓			✓	
Reflective	✓	✓		✓		✓			✓	
Ethical sensitivity	✓	✓		✓		✓			✓	✓
Accountability	✓			✓	✓		✓	✓		✓
Confidence	✓	✓					✓		✓	✓

Activity 12.3: Critical thinking and decision-making (page 217)

(i) NMC Standards (Table 12.1) which, on the case study evidence, were not fully complied with by one of the nurses:

- *Listen to people and respond to their preferences and concerns* (p4).
- *Make sure that people's physical, social and psychological needs are assessed and responded to* (p5).
- *Make sure that you get properly informed consent and document it before carrying out any action* (p6).
- *Respect people's right to privacy and confidentiality* (p6).
- *Recognise when people are anxious or in distress and respond compassionately and politely* (p5).
- *Act in partnership with those receiving care, helping them to access relevant health and social care, information and support when they need it* (p5).
- *Gather and reflect on feedback from a variety of sources, using it to improve your practice and performance* (p8).

(ii) Mitigating factors that may have contributed to this non-compliance:

- Workload pressure and weight of responsibility in ensuring routine tasks performed as scheduled.
- The consultant informed Rosemary that giving her an enema was a necessary preparatory procedure.
- The radiologist was depending on nurses giving Rosemary the enema to get a clear picture.
- The sister may have thought being firm with Rosemary was the best way to ensure she co-operated.
- She believed it was in Rosemary's best interests to have the enema to help diagnose her problem.
- She may not have been given sufficient staff development or training opportunities to update skills.
- She may possibly have personal health and wellbeing issues of her own which impact on her work.
- She may not have updated her knowledge regarding the revised version of *The Code* (NMC, 2015).

(iii) Staff might be helped to comply with NMC Standards in future by:

- Feedback about their performance in relation to apparent non-compliance with the NMC *Code*.
- Reading *The Code* (NMC, 2015), being conversant with its contents and referring to it regularly.
- Applying PERSON clinical decision-making evaluation tool incorporating key NMC Standards.
- Ensuring there is an adequate allocation of staff and an appropriate skill mix in clinical areas.
- Providing staff development and training opportunities to update knowledge and skills.
- Supervision in which problems and professional development issues can be identified and resolved.
- Staff meetings to exchange ideas, consider alternative perspectives and support each other.

(iv) Consequences of non-compliance with *The Code*:

- In the case study, the consequences for Rosemary were that the sister: did not listen or respond to her concerns; did not assess and respond to her psychological needs; did not gain informed consent from Rosemary to carry out the enema; did not respect her right to privacy and confidentiality; was not compassionate or polite when Rosemary became distressed; did not act in partnership with Rosemary; and did not appear to reflect on how she had upset Rosemary.
- If this pattern of behaviour is repeated with other patients it is likely their sense of wellbeing will also be adversely affected. If one is made aware of such criticisms, it presents an opportunity to reflect and learn better ways of communicating with patients and respecting their right to self-determination. Where nurses acknowledge weaknesses, identify areas for improvement and remediate what was lacking in their behaviour, the experience contributes to their professional development.
- If we are made aware that we are not meeting NMC Standards and choose to ignore it, we will be placing our registration as nurses in jeopardy. We could be reported to the NMC who will be duty bound to investigate any allegations of professional misconduct in order to protect the public.

Further reading

Ellis, P (2016) *Evidence-based practice in nursing* (3rd edn). London: Sage/Learning Matters.

Chapter 7, Clinical decision-making in evidence-based nursing, applies PERSON to evaluate a case study.

Howatson-Jones, L, Standing, M and Roberts, S (2015) *Patient assessment and care planning in nursing* (2nd edn). London: Sage/Learning Matters.

Chapter 10, Patient assessment and decision-making, applies PERSON to evaluate a child pathway case study.

Useful websites

www.mencap.org.uk/get-involved/here-i-am?gclid=CNSCkdvZ39ACFcq97QodF04KNA

This page on Mencap's website links to a film in which Casey Rochelle (Aka DJ Dude), a self-confessed lover of life and music, who also happens to have Down's syndrome and autism, uses his DJ skills to remix a recording by an unidentified academic in 1968 who is saying: *There is no reason to feel guilty about putting a Down's syndrome child away. True guilt arises only from an offence against a person and a Down's is not a person.* After Casey has finished editing the recording it is considerably shorter and has a completely different meaning, as follows: 'DOWN'S IS A PERSON!'

Glossary

accountability in clinical decision-making being answerable to patients, public, employers, the NMC and the law for the consequences of actions, and having to explain, justify or defend your decisions.

clinical decision-making applies clinical judgement to select the best possible evidence-based option to control risks and address patients' needs in high quality care for which you are accountable.

clinical judgement informed opinion (using intuition, reflection and critical thinking) that relates observation and assessment of patients to identifying and evaluating alternative nursing options.

cognitive continuum judgement ranging from intuitive hunches to critical analysis that is tailored to the constantly changing nature of the clinical demands and health problems that we deal with.

collaborative decision-making consulting with patients, relatives, nurses, mentors, managers and other health professionals or agencies in order to inform relevant patient-centred decisions.

confidence in decision-making self-assurance from previous experience or achievements and professional assurance (respecting confidentiality, applying evidence-based practice) to inspire patients to trust you to help them and enable you to explain, justify and defend your decisions.

critical incidents events that have a significant impact on you, prompting you to reflect on them.

critical thinking questioning one's own and others' assumptions, addressing gaps in knowledge to achieve aims, challenging illogical or unethical beliefs or practice, evaluating the strength of available evidence and presenting a logical, evidence-based argument and defending it when challenged.

embedded knowledge information cues in clinical practice requiring keen observation to detect.

embodied knowledge subconscious accumulation of personal experience drawn on in intuition.

espoused theories concepts, academic knowledge derived from formal learning in university.

ethical sensitivity in decision-making applying ethical principles (do not harm, actions beneficial, respect freedom of choice, fairness to all); for example, inform patients and obtain consent to care, respect confidentiality, break 'bad news' compassionately and discuss treatment dilemmas.

evidence any kind of information that is used to support reasoning, problem solving, clinical judgement and decision-making, including observations, feedback, policy, theory and research.

evidence-based practice   never being satisfied that you 'know it all', and using critical thinking skills to continually search, access, evaluate and apply the most relevant up-to-date sources and types of information to guide clinical judgement/decision-making in giving high quality care.

experience and intuition in clinical decision-making   recognising similarities and differences between current and previous situations and being guided by what seemed effective before (and learning from any earlier mistakes) or realising you lack the necessary experience to make a decision.

hermeneutic phenomenology   a method by which a researcher seeks to elicit a person's perceptions of interacting with others and how they make sense of their lived experience without imposing one's own agenda.

holistic   associated with the phrase 'the whole is greater than the sum of its parts'. When applied to healthcare it involves understanding patients' biological, psychological, social and spiritual needs, and caring for the whole person rather than focusing solely on a health problem.

Matrix model   comprising of ten perceptions of decision-making and ten conceptions of nursing, identified by nurses in a phenomenological longitudinal research study, describing unique nature of nurses' decisions.

nursing   promoting health and wellbeing, relief from suffering, recovery from illness or injury, adaptation to disability and dignity in facing death in patient-centred care, applying bio-psycho-social-spiritual knowledge, skills and ethical values to safe, effective judgement, decisions and evidence-based practice.

nursing theory   philosophy or model-defining interrelationships between concepts of 'humans/environment/health/nursing' to explain values, vital knowledge or skills and aim of nurses' role.

observation in clinical decision-making   continuous use of senses (sight, hearing, touch or smell) to assess patients' bio-psycho-social-spiritual wellbeing, check if they need assistance, monitor vital signs, review results of investigations, record response to treatment and report concerns.

patient/person-centred care   tailoring care that is relevant and responsive to a patient's needs and concerns by identifying their preferences, explaining options and enabling them to make informed decisions about the care they wish to receive.

'PERSON' evaluation tool   a new universal framework to question, evaluate and guide nursing and midwifery decisions/interventions in the six key areas, namely: Patient-centred/Evidence-based/Risks assessed and managed/Safe and effective delivery of care/Outcomes benefit patient/Nursing and midwifery strengths and weaknesses.

prioritising in decision-making   applying risk assessment and management to target care: on those with life-threatening illness or injury before others; on a patient's urgent needs before non-urgent needs; on health promotion for vulnerable groups; and on avoiding causing harm to patients in healthcare settings.

problem solving   dissatisfaction with current situation prompts the use of critical thinking skills to systematically assess and identify the problem, plan and implement action and evaluate the outcome.

reflective decision-making   review events as they occur (reflection-in-action) to identify and choose best option or to review past (reflection-on-action) for insights to inform future practice.

reflexivity critical self-examination of the logic and evidence for what we think is true by being open about our potential biases, assuming our interpretations may be wrong and testing them.

standardised clinical decision-making apply NHS Trust policies, procedures and agreed care plans plus evidence-based (NICE) clinical guidelines and assessment tools to guide nursing interventions.

systematic clinical decision-making use of critical thinking and problem-solving skills to identify/assess problems, set goals/make plans, deliver nursing care and evaluate outcome (revise as needed).

theories-in-use assumptions, custom and practice derived from informal work-based learning.

theory–practice gap mismatch between what nurses are taught and what they actually do.

References

Aked, J, Marks, N, Cordon, C and Thompson, S (2008) *Five ways to well being: a report presented to the Foresight Project on communicating the evidence base for improving people's well-being*. New Economic Foundation. Available at: www.businessballs.com/freespecialresources/Five_Ways_to_Well-being-NEF.pdf.

ALC (Alcohol Learning Centre) (2016) *Identification and brief advice tool*. London: ALC. Available at: www.alcohollearningcentre.org.uk/Topics/Latest/Identification-and-Brief-Advice-Tool-2016-revised-April-2016.

Alfaro-LeFevre, R (2013) *Applying nursing process: the foundation for clinical reasoning* (8th edn). Philadelphia, PA: Lippincott Williams & Wilkins.

Argyris, C and Schön, D (1974) *Theory in practice: increasing personal effectiveness*. Boston, MA: Addison Wesley.

Babor, TF, Higgins-Biddle, JC, Saunders, JB and Monteiro, MG (2001) *AUDIT: The Alcohol Use Disorders Identification Test* (2nd edn). Geneva: WHO.

Bach, A and Grant, S (2015) *Communication and interpersonal skills for nurses* (3rd edn). London: Sage/Learning Matters.

BBC (2010) *Tetraplegic man's life support turned off by mistake*. Available at: www.bbc.co.uk/news/uk-england-wiltshire-11595485.

Beauchamp, T and Childress, J (1989) *Principles of biomedical ethics*. Oxford: Oxford University Press.

Beck, J (2011) *CBT: basics and beyond* (2nd edn). New York: Guilford Press.

Benner, P (1984) *From novice to expert*. Menlo Park, CA: Addison-Wesley.

Bloom, B (1956) *Taxonomy of educational objectives: Book 1. The cognitive domain*. London: Longman.

Campbell, H, Hotchkiss, R, Bradshaw, N and Porteous, M (1998) Integrated care pathways. *BMJ (British Medical Journal)*, 316(7125): 133–137.

Cancer Research UK (2016) *Lifetime risk of cancer*. Available at: www.cancerresearchuk.org/health-professional/cancer-statistics/risk/lifetime-risk#heading-Zero.

Chambers (2016) *Chambers 21st Century Dictionary*. London: Hodder and Stoughton. Available at: www.chambers.co.uk/book/the-chambers-dictionary.

Clark, J (2006) 30th anniversary commentary on Henderson V (1978) *The concept of nursing. Journal of Advanced Nursing*, 3: 113–130.

Corcoran-Perry, S and Narayan, S (1995) Clinical decision-making. In: Snyder, M and Mirr, MP (eds) *Advanced nursing practice*. New York: Springer.

Cullum, N, Ciliska, D, Haynes, B and Marks, S (eds) (2007) *Evidence-based nursing: an introduction*. Oxford: Blackwell.

DH (Department of Health) (2000) *The NHS Plan*. London: HMSO.

DH (2006) Expert Patients Programme. London: HMSO.

DH (2008a) *High quality care for all: NHS Next Step Review final report.* London: HMSO.

DH (2008b) *Human rights in healthcare: a framework for local action* (2nd edn). London: HMSO.

DH (2012a) *Compassion in practice: nursing, midwifery and care staff – our vision and strategy.* Available at: www.england.nhs.uk/wp-content/uploads/2012/12/compassion-in-practice.pdf.

DH (2012b) *Liberating the NHS: no decision about me, without me.* London: HMSO.

DH (2013a) *The NHS Constitution.* London: HMSO.

DH (2013b) *National Early Warning Score.* National Clinical Guideline No. 1. National Clinical Effectiveness Committee. London: HMSO.

DH (2016a) *National Child Measurement Programme: operational guidance.* London: HMSO.

DH (2016b) *NHS Outcomes Framework 2016 to 2017.* London: HMSO.

Dyer, L (2015) A review of the impact of the human rights in healthcare programme in England and Wales. *Health and Human Rights Journal,* 17(2): 111–122.

Ellis, A and Dryden, W (2007) *The practice of rational emotive behaviour therapy* (2nd edn). New York: Springer.

Ellis, P (2016) *Evidence-based practice in nursing* (3rd edn). London: Sage/Learning Matters.

Fawcett, J and DeSanto-Madeya, S (2012) *Contemporary nursing knowledge: analysis and evaluation of nursing models and theories* (3rd edn). Philadelphia, PA: FA Davies.

Francis Report (2013) *The Mid Staffordshire NHS Foundation Trust Public Inquiry.* Available at: www.midstaffs publicinquiry.com/report.

Gardner, H (1983) *Frames of mind: the theory of multiple intelligences.* New York: Basic Books.

Gawande, A (2011) *The checklist manifesto: how to get things right.* London: Profile Books.

Gibbs, G (1988) *Learning by doing: a guide to teaching and learning methods.* London: Further Education Unit.

Gibney, P (2006) The double-bind theory: still crazy making after all these years. *Psychotherapy in Australia,* 12(3): 48–55. Available at: www.psychotherapy.com.au/fileadmin/site_files/pdfs/TheDoubleBind Theory.pdf

Gonzalez, J and Wagenaar, R (2003) *Tuning educational structures in Europe: final report pilot project – phase 1.* Bilbao: University of Deusto.

Griffith, JW and Christensen, PJ (1982) *Nursing process: application of theories, frameworks and models.* St Louis, MO: Mosby.

Griffith, R and Tengnah, C (2017) *Law and professional issues in nursing* (4th edn). London: Sage/Learning Matters.

Hammond, KR (1996) *Human judgement and social policy: irreducible uncertainty, inevitable error, unavoidable injustice.* New York: Oxford University Press.

Haynes, AB, Weisner, TG, Berry, WR et al. (2009) A surgical safety checklist to reduce morbidity and mortality in a global population. *New England Journal of Medicine,* 360: 491–499.

Henderson, V (1966) *The nature of nursing.* New York: Macmillan.

Hernanz-Schulman, M (2003) Infantile hypertrophic pyloric stenosis. *Radiology,* 227: 319–331.

Heron, J (2001) *Helping the client: a creative practical guide* (5th edn). London: Sage.

Higgs, J and Titchen, A (2001) *Practice knowledge and expertise.* Oxford: Butterworth Heinemann.

HSCIC (Health and Social Care Information Centre) (2016) *Statistics on alcohol.* Available at: www.content.digital.nhs.uk/catalogue/PUB20999/alc-eng-2016-rep.pdf.

HSE (Health and Safety Executive) (2011) *Five steps to risk assessment.* Available at: www.hse.gov.uk/risk/fivesteps.htm.

ICN (International Council of Nurses) (2009) *ICN framework of competencies for the nurse specialist.* Geneva: ICN.

Jasper, M, Rosser, M and Mooney, G (eds) (2013) *Professional development, reflection and decision-making in nursing and healthcare.* Oxford: Blackwell.

Johns, C (2010) *Guided reflection: a narrative approach to advancing professional practice* (2nd edn). Chichester: Wiley-Blackwell.

Keogh Report (2013) *Review into the quality of care and treatment provided by 14 hospital trusts in England: NHS England.* Available at: www.nhs.uk/NHSEngland/bruce-keogh-review/Documents/outcomes/keogh-review-final-report.pdf.

Kipling, R (1902) I keep six honest serving men (from R Kipling, *The Elephant's Child – Just So Stories*). Available at: www.kipling.org.uk/poems_serving.htm.

Kolb, DA (1984) *Experiential learning.* Englewood Cliffs, NJ: Prentice Hall.

Lam, A (2000) Tacit knowledge, organizational learning and societal institutions: an integrated framework. *Organizational Studies,* 21: 487–513.

Leininger, M (1985) Transcultural nursing care: diversity and universality. *Nursing and Health Care,* 6: 209–212.

Melnyk, BM and Fineout-Overholt, E (2014) *Evidence-based practice in nursing and healthcare: a guide to best practice* (3rd edn). Philadelphia, PA: Walters Kluwer/Lippincott Williams and Wilkins.

Middleton, S, Barnett, J and Reeves, D (2001) What is an integrated care pathway? *Evidence Based Medicine,* 3(3): 1–7.

Moule, P (2015) *Making sense of research in nursing, health and social care* (5th edn). London: Sage.

NHS (2010) What's your BMI? Available at: www.nhs.uk/LiveWell/loseweight/Pages/BodyMassIndex.aspx.

NHS England (2014) *The Five Year Forward View.* Available at: www.england.nhs.uk/publications/ourwork/futurenhs.

NICE (National Institute for Health and Care Excellence) (2007a) *How to change practice: understand, identify and overcome barriers to change.* London: NICE.

NICE (2007b) *Acutely ill patients in hospital: recognition and response to acute illness in hospital.* London: NICE.

NICE (2009) *Depression: the treatment and management of depression in adults.* Clinical Guideline CG90. London: NICE.

NICE (2010a) *Alcohol use disorders: preventing harmful drinking.* Public Health Guidance PHG24. London: NICE.

NICE (2010b) *Chest pain of recent onset.* Clinical Guideline CG95. London: NICE.

NICE (2011) *Generalised anxiety disorder and panic disorder (with or without agoraphobia) in adults.* Clinical Guideline CG113. London: NICE.

NICE (2012) *Patient experience in adult NHS services: improving the experience of care for people using adult NHS services.* Clinical Guideline CG138. London: NICE.

NICE (2013) *Embedding shared decision making in 32 national teams.* London: NICE.

NICE (2015a) *Violence and aggression: short-term management in mental health, health and community settings.* London: NICE.

NICE (2015b) *Challenging behaviour and learning difficulties.* Guideline NG11. London: NICE.

Nightingale, F (1860) *Notes on nursing: what it is and what it is not.* New York: Appleton.

NMC (Nursing and Midwifery Council) (2010) *Standards for pre-registration nursing education.* London: NMC.

NMC (2015) *The Code: professional standards of practice and behaviour for nurses and midwives.* London: NMC.

NMC (2016) *Nursing and Midwifery Council annual fitness to practise report 2015–2016.* London: NMC.

Olver, K (2007) *Ten critical de-escalation skills.* Available at: www.populararticles.com/article45613.html.

ONS (Office for National Statistics) (2016a) *Deaths registered in England and Wales, 2015.* Available at: www.ons.gov.uk/peoplepopulationandcommunity/birthsdeathsandmarriages/deaths/datasets/deathregistrations summarytablesenglandandwalesreferencetables. 2015: Current [xls (340.0kB)]. Table 2 Deaths by age, sex and underlying cause, 2015 registrations. U509, V01-Y89 External causes of morbidity and mortality. V01-V89 Land transport accidents.

ONS (2016b) *Overview of the UK population: February 2016.* London: HMSO.

ORCIC (Office of the Regulator of Community Interest Companies) and DBIS (Department for Business Innovation and Skills) (2013) *Case study: the Expert Patients Programme.* London: ORCIC and DBIS. Available at: www.gov.uk/government/case-studies/the-expert-patients-programme.

Orem, D (1980) *Nursing: concepts of practice.* New York: McGraw-Hill.

Parse, RR (1992) Human becoming: Parse's theory of nursing. *Nursing Science Quarterly,* 5(1): 35–42.

Peplau, H (1952) *Interpersonal relations in nursing.* New York: Putman and Sons.

Powell, H and Murray, G (2004) Staff perceptions of community learning disability nurses' role. *Nursing Times,* 100(19): 40.

Proctor, B (1986) Supervision: a co-operative exercise in accountability. In: Marken, M and Payne, M (eds) *Enabling and ensuring: supervision in practice.* Leicester: National Youth Bureau, Council for Education and Training in Youth and Community Work.

Pronovost, P, Needham, D, Berenholtz, S et al. (2006) An intervention to reduce catheter-related bloodstream infections in the ICU. *New England Journal of Medicine,* 355: 2725–2732.

RCN (Royal College of Nursing) (2010) *Principles of nursing practice.* London: RCN.

RCN (2014a) *Defining nursing.* London: RCN.

RCN (2014b) *Learning from the past – setting out the future: developing learning disability nursing in the United Kingdom.* London: RCN.

RCP (Royal College of Physicians) (2015) *National Early Warning Score (NEWS).* London: RCP.

Reed, S (2015) *Successful professional portfolios for nursing students* (2nd edn). London: Sage/Learning Matters.

Reinharz, S (1997) Who am I? The need for a variety of selves in the field. In: Hertz, R (ed.) *Reflexivity and voice.* Thousand Oaks, CA: Sage.

Rogers, EM (1962) *Diffusion of innovations.* Glencoe: Free Press.

Rolfe, G, Segrott, J and Jordon, S (2008) Tensions and contradictions in nurses' perspectives of evidence-based practice. *Journal of Nursing Management,* 16(4): 440–451.

Roper, N, Logan, WW and Tierney, AJ (2000) *The Roper–Logan–Tierney model of nursing: based on activities of living.* Edinburgh: Churchill Livingstone.

Roy, C (1980) *Introduction to nursing: an adaptation model.* Englewood Cliffs, NJ: Prentice Hall.

Rycroft-Malone, J, Seers, K, Titchen, A et al. (2004) What counts as evidence-based practice? *Journal of Advanced Nursing,* 47: 81–90.

Schön, DA (1983) *The reflective practitioner.* New York: Basic Books.

Snyder, M (1995) Advanced practice within a nursing paradigm. In: Snyder, M and Mirr, MP (eds) *Advanced nursing practice.* New York: Springer.

Standing, M (1999) Developing a Supportive/Challenging and Reflective/Competency Education (SCARCE) mentoring model and discussing its relevance to nurse education. *Mentoring and Tutoring,* 6(3): 3–17.

Standing, M (2005) *Perceptions of clinical decision-making on a developmental journey from student to staff nurse.* Unpublished PhD Thesis. Canterbury: University of Kent.

Standing, M (2007) Clinical decision-making skills on the developmental journey from student to registered nurse: a longitudinal inquiry. *Journal of Advanced Nursing,* 60(3): 257–269.

Standing, M (2008) Nine modes of practice in a revised cognitive continuum. *Journal of Advanced Nursing,* 62(1): 124–134.

Standing, M (2009) A new critical framework for applying hermeneutic phenomenology. *Nurse Researcher,* 16(4): 20–30.

Standing, M (2010a) Perceptions of clinical decision-making: a matrix model. In: Standing, M (ed.) *Clinical judgement and decision-making: nursing and interprofessional healthcare.* Maidenhead: McGraw-Hill Education/Open University Press.

Standing, M (2010b) Cognitive continuum theory: nine modes of practice. In: Standing, M (ed.) *Clinical judgement and decision-making: nursing and interprofessional healthcare.* Maidenhead: McGraw-Hill Education/Open University Press.

Standing, M and Standing, MRJ (2010) Reflexive-pragmatism: logic, practicality, rigour and relevance. In: Standing, M (ed.) *Clinical judgement and decision-making: nursing and interprofessional healthcare.* Maidenhead: McGraw-Hill Education/Open University Press.

SJA et al. (St John Ambulance, St Andrews Ambulance Association and British Red Cross Society) (2016) *First aid manual* (10th edn). London: Dorling Kindersley.

Trenoweth, S, Docherty, T, Franks, J and Pearce, R (2011) *Nursing and mental health care: an introduction for all fields of practice.* Exeter: Learning Matters.

Trower, P, Casey, A and Dryden, W (1988) *Cognitive-behavioural counselling in action.* London: Sage.

Watson, J (1988) *Nursing: human science and human care.* New York: National League for Nursing.

WHO (World Health Organization) (1948) *Official records of the World Health Organization.* Geneva: WHO.

WHO (2009) *Surgical safety checklist.* Geneva: WHO.

Yates, A (2016) The risks and benefits of suprapubic catheters. *Nursing Times,* 112(6/7): 19–22.

Yura, H and Walsh, MB (1973) *The nursing process.* New York: Appleton-Century-Crofts.

Index

Made in the USA
Lexington, KY
09 June 2017